For Women Only

FOR WOMEN ONLY

A Revolutionary Guide to Overcoming Sexual Dysfunction and Reclaiming Your Sex Life

Jennifer Berman, M.D., and Laura Berman, Ph.D.

with Elisabeth Bumiller

HENRY HOLT AND COMPANY • NEW YORK

Henry Holt and Company, LLC
Publishers since 1866
115 West 18th Street
New York, New York 10011
Henry Holt® is a registered trademark of Henry Holt and Company, LLC.

Library of Congress Cataloging-in-Publication Data
Berman, Jennifer, M.D.
    For women only: a revolutionary guide to overcoming sexual dysfunction
and reclaiming your sex life / Jennifer Berman and Laura Berman, with
Elisabeth Bumiller.
        p.   cm.
    Includes bibliographical references and index.
    ISBN 0-8050-6405-2 (hb)
    1. Women—Sexual behavior.   2. Women—Health and hygiene.
3. Hygiene, Sexual.   4. Sex instruction for women.   5. Sexual disorders.
I. Berman, Laura.   II. Bumiller, Elisabeth.   III. Title.

RG103 .B465 2001
613.9'54—dc21   00-049901

Henry Holt books are available for special promotions
and premiums. For details contact:
Director, Special Markets.
First Edition 2001
Designed by Fearn Cutler

Printed in the United States of America
1   3   5   7   9   10   8   6   4   2

To our parents:
our father for teaching us that nothing is impossible and
our mother for empowering us to believe it to be true

A Note to Readers

This book is intended to help you improve your sexual health, but it is not a substitute for a physician's or psychotherapist's advice and treatment. Please consult your own medical doctor or psychotherapist before embarking on any of these treatments.

Contents

Introduction

This is, at heart, a book about the female sexual response. We believe that what women and their partners learn here will eliminate much anguish and despair and help them enjoy more sexually satisfied lives. *For Women Only* also reflects the enormous change in the treatment of women's sexual problems in the last three years. Our book grew out of this exploding new field, and we are privileged to have played a part. Female sexual dysfunction is at last on the table—a recognized and often treatable disorder, which affects the general health and quality of life of millions of women around the world.

What you read here is based directly on our work when we were codirectors of the Women's Sexual Health Clinic at Boston University Medical Center. Thanks to the help of our mentor and role model, Dr. Irwin Goldstein, the pioneer and leader in the field of male erectile dysfunction, this clinic was an enormous success.

We are sisters and started the clinic together, which was the realization of a longtime dream. We had talked for years about the possibility, particularly as Jennifer, a surgeon and anatomist and one of the few women urologists in a nearly all-male field, became convinced that women could benefit from the same medical attention to sexual problems that was given to men. Laura, a sex therapist and psychotherapist heavily schooled in anthropology, enthusiastically supported Jennifer's views.

We opened our doors in the summer of 1998 and have not caught our breath since. The clinic was among the first in the country to offer comprehensive treatment, both physiological and psychological, for women suffering from sexual dysfunction. We have made it clear from the beginning that while we could learn a tremendous amount from the treatment of male sexual dysfunction, we were not going to subscribe to the initial efforts of many physicians to define "female impotence" in masculine terms. We treat women with female sexual dysfunction in terms of four newly classified categories—hypoactive sexual desire disorder, sexual arousal disorder, orgasmic disorder, and sexual pain disorders—as well as a wide variety of other problems. We also offer sex therapy, couples therapy, educational counseling, medical treatment, and surgery. We answer frequently asked questions: What is orgasm? How can I enhance my sex life? Am I normal? How can I get my partner to fulfill my sexual needs? Our work is exciting and rewarding. With new medical technology and medications as well as existing psychotherapy treatments, women now have more options than ever before.

Clearly, help is needed for women as much as men. Studies estimate that more than half the women over age 40 in the United States have sexual complaints. In early 1999, the National Health and Social Life Survey published in the *Journal of the American Medical Association* released a report showing sexual problems to be even more widespread: the survey found that 43 percent of American women, young and old, suffer from some sexual dysfunction—a significantly higher percentage than that of men, who suffer at a rate of 31 percent.

And yet for most of this century doctors have dismissed women's sexual complaints as either psychological or emotional. In the nineteenth century, the Victorians believed that "good" women had no sexual desires at all. Even now, in our supposedly enlightened era, it is still shocking for us to hear how many doctors, female as well as male, tell their female patients that their problems are emotional, relational, or due to fatigue from child rearing or their busy jobs, and that they should take care of their problems on their own. Many doctors tell older women that these are not real problems at all, just something to accept as a normal part of aging. This is particularly true of older women, although women of all ages have reported this to us.

We hope this book will serve as an antidote to what women have heard for decades. The problem is not "just in your head." You are not crazy, or alone, or fated never to have an orgasm or feel sexual again. Of course, we don't dismiss the importance of psychological factors. But in our experience with our patients, who come from all over the United States and the world, and from all age groups and cultural backgrounds, most problems tend to have both medical and emotional roots, and feed on each other. Our goal in this comprehensive handbook on sexual health is to help the whole woman.

In our clinical work we have always worked as a team. Jennifer conducts the medical part of our patient evaluation and treatment. She is also in charge of our laboratory research, including a recently completed study funded by the American Foundation for Urologic Disease on the smooth muscle function of the vagina and clitoris. This research helped us better understand the mechanisms underlying female sexual arousal responses. Laura is the clinic's psychotherapist. She has a Ph.D. in health education and therapy, with a speciality in human sexuality. She interviews and evaluates patients both before and after Jennifer sees them, and determines if they have emotional problems or relational conflicts that require treatment on a longer basis. Laura helps them get a sense of the larger picture of their lives, and provides ongoing therapy to individuals, couples, and families if needed.

Both of us feel that women's sexual complaints are still neglected by the medical establishment, and that many of the same health problems that cause erectile dysfunction in men, such as diabetes, high blood pressure, and high cholesterol, as well as many medications used to treat these conditions, can cause sexual dysfunction in women. Most women also experience diminished sexual responsiveness and loss of libido at the onset of menopause, and many have sexual complaints after hysterectomy or other pelvic surgery. Although drug companies have worked for years to treat male impotence, they are only just beginning to recognize female sexual dysfunction as a medical problem. Even female sexual anatomy is not completely known or understood. It was not until 1998 that an Australian urologist, Helen O'Connell, discovered that the clitoris is twice as large and more complex than generally described in medical texts.

The fact remains that there has been a great deal of psychological research but almost no medical research into the sexual response of women since the groundbreaking work of

William H. Masters and Virginia E. Johnson in their laboratory in St. Louis, Missouri, in 1966. Masters and Johnson
were the first to describe the physical changes in the vagina
during sexual arousal, which they observed and filmed in
volunteers with a small vaginal probe and a camera attachment. We have begun where Masters and Johnson left off.

We have adapted the more sophisticated technology of
our day: pH probes to measure lubrication; a balloon device
to evaluate the ability of the vagina to relax and dilate; vi-
bratory and heat and cold sensation measures of the external and internal genitalia; and high frequency Doppler
imaging, or ultrasound, to measure blood flow to the vagina
and clitoris during arousal. Ultrasound, which has been
widely available since the 1970s, has never before been used
to evaluate genital blood flow when a woman is sexually
aroused. Currently, even more sophisticated instruments are
being developed to evaluate female sexual arousal, response,
and function. These include probes to measure vaginal, clitoral, and nipple sensation, and computerized equipment to
measure vaginal anatomy and physiology in the office. MRI,
or magnetic resonance imaging, is even being used to determine what areas of the brain are responsible for arousal and
orgasm.

One of our most important findings is that a physical
problem—a decrease in blood flow to the vagina and uterus,
perhaps as a result of aging, hysterectomy, or other pelvic or
vascular surgery—may be a cause of a diminished sexual
response just as diminished blood flow may affect male sexuality. Some women have sexual complaints after hysterectomies and often are told by doctors that they are simply
depressed. We believe that in some cases injury to the nerves
and blood supply to the genital area may be the cause or be

contributing to the problem. Jennifer is in fact developing the same nerve-sparing pelvic surgery for women as is available for men who undergo prostate surgery. Furthermore, we are beginning to realize the important role testosterone plays in female sexual function and dysfunction.

Our goal in this book is to arm women with the information they need about their bodies and sexual response and to provide them with a full spectrum of options for treatment. Our hope is that women will take this book to their doctors, give it to their partners, or share it with other women. It is written without jargon, by women, for women. Clearly, the options will continue to grow as more research is done in this field, and it is also our plan to update women with the latest information.

We are in a new era of women's sexual health—perhaps feminism's next frontier. Sex is central to intimacy, to who we are, to our emotional well-being and quality of life. Doctors have assumed for years that as long as a woman is able to have intercourse without pain, all is well. That is simply not the case. The fact that sexual education has rarely been a part of physicians' education and training has further aggravated the problem. Most male physicians have only their personal life experiences to help them understand female sexuality. We hope that this book will also help bridge that gap and encourage early education in sexuality for physicians and health care professionals in training and help educate those currently in practice.

It is high time for women to receive the same attention as men, and to demand treatment, not only for pain, but to increase their sexual pleasure.

CHAPTER ONE

Our Approach to Women's Sexual Health

When Nicole arrived at our clinic early one December morning with complaints that she had no interest in sex, we could see how nervous she was.* But then, almost every woman who walks through our door is a little frightened at first. It's the normal reaction, since sex is not normally addressed openly in any setting, much less a doctor's office. Our immediate task is to put our patients at ease. They're always relieved to learn that many other women share the very same problems, that they're not abnormal or alone. A lot of women will tell us that they are embarrassed that their sexuality is so important to them, and that they feel they aren't entitled to feeling sexual because they are older. The younger women often say they are unable or afraid to talk to their partners about their sexual problems. These attitudes reflect the long-standing pressure on women to acknowledge sex as a basic part of their lives but not to feel entitled to an optimum response.

Nicole, a 40-year-old bank loan officer from Kentucky,

*Like all patients in this book, Nicole's name has been changed to protect her privacy.

learned about us from an article in a women's magazine about female sexual dysfunction. Like a lot of our patients, she had finally decided that her problems were important enough to take time off from work and travel a long way to see us. "It's been pretty stressful," she told Laura. "I feel bad for my partner." Other patients are referred by their gynecologists, primary care doctors, or internists, or hear about us by word of mouth. Others are interested in trying Viagra, which we have successfully prescribed to a number of female patients. Some of those patients have taken part in our Viagra trial, one of the earliest studies of the drug's effects on women. (For the results of our Viagra study, and information about Jennifer's research on vaginal and clitoral tissue, see pages 18 to 20 at the end of this chapter.)

When Nicole had called to make her appointment, she spoke briefly to Laura. During these initial phone calls, many women break down and cry out of frustration from having dealt with this issue alone for so long. Others cry from relief that someone is finally listening to them. Nicole was more matter-of-fact. Laura asked her a little about herself and to describe her problem. Then, as Laura does with all of our patients, she told Nicole what to expect during her upcoming visit to the clinic: Nicole would first talk to Laura and then be evaluated by Jennifer. Following her medical evaluation, she would then undergo our physical testing in a private examination room. We explained that in order to fully evaluate her arousal problem, if one existed, and determine its cause (for example, hormone levels, low genital blood flow, decreased genital sensation, or low vaginal lubrication), we would need to evaluate her, as best we could, under conditions of sexual arousal. Her physiological sexual responses would then be measured. Although this situation does not reproduce what happens in the privacy of one's own home, it does provide us with a lot of useful information.

We evaluated Nicole over a period of two days. On the first day we evaluated her baseline sexual response without medication. On the second day, the evaluations were repeated after she took Viagra.

What happened after that, during Nicole's two days at our clinic, will tell you a lot about who we are and how we work. We also hope that Nicole's case, and those we've included here of two other patients, Maria and Paula, will clarify what our patients tell us is a professional, caring, and very positive experience.

The first thing Nicole did in our office was fill out several short questionnaires asking about her sexual functioning over the previous month. These forms, used by all of our patients, ask for basic medical and relationship information. They also ask them to rate their sexual desire, their ability to become aroused, their level of lubrication, any sensations they feel in their genital area during sex, any feelings of numbness, their ability to reach orgasm, whether they experience any pain during intercourse, how satisfied they are with their partner's stimulation, and their feelings of emotional intimacy during sex.

After Nicole completed the forms, she went in to see Laura for a 45-minute psychosexual evaluation. Laura uses an assessment model she created called the Biopsychosocial Sexual Evaluation System (BSES), through which she is able to get an initial impression of not only the sexual history of the patient, but the source of the sexual function complaints as well. After these sessions, often the first time that the patient has talked to anyone at length about her difficulties, Laura can identify red flags that signal the need for further evaluation and potential treatment, either physical or emotional. A course of action, both medical and psychotherapeutic, can begin to be developed based on the findings.

When Laura first asked Nicole to describe as specifically as possible her problem and why she had come, Nicole responded that not only had she lost desire, but also that she had trouble with vaginal lubrication and could not reach orgasm when she did have sex. She traced her problems to laser surgery for skin cancer of the vulva that she had undergone three years earlier. Nicole told Laura that she had at one time enjoyed sex enormously—"I remember having orgasms and being real wet"—but since her cancer surgery "it hasn't been anything like it was before." Nicole also told Laura that she was on Paxil, an SSRI (selective seratonin reuptake inhibitor) antidepressant, which can cause a loss of libido, vaginal dryness, and difficulty in reaching orgasm. (For more about the effects of antidepressants on sexual function, see chapter 4.)

Because early childhood experiences can impact on sexuality later in life, Laura next asked Nicole about her early childhood and adolescence, her attitudes toward sex when she was growing up, her parents' attitudes, and her past sexual experiences. Like many of the women we see, Nicole said she had been raised to believe that premarital sex was wrong, and that her brother had always told her that "if you had sex, a guy wouldn't respect you." She first had intercourse at the age of 19 with a boyfriend and described the experience as physically painful, although she began to enjoy sex a few years later with a different partner. She apologetically said that sex was always easier for her after a few drinks—"I move better, probably, and I'm looser"—and that in general it was hard to let herself go without alcohol. Nicole also told Laura that she had tried masturbation, but had never used it to reach orgasm, and was afraid to try a vibrator. "I always heard if you used a vibrator," she said, repeating something we hear all the time, "that you wouldn't want a man." Other women worry—wrongly—that they will become dependent on a vibrator or be unable to become aroused or reach orgasm without it.

Nicole's words were strikingly but typically full of self-reproach. She was blaming herself for her problems. It didn't help that they were also upsetting her relationship with her partner. "A lot of times I don't reach orgasm, which makes him feel inferior," she said. Her partner, Nicole said, was now having trouble getting an erection or maintaining one. But she also admitted that she sometimes resented him for expecting that it was "my job" to arouse him. "Sometimes I really don't like to work to get it hard," she said. At one point, as Nicole cataloged her problems with her partner, she quietly wept.

Afterward, Laura recounted the session to Jennifer and summarized the important psychological factors and problems with the relationship that could be contributing to Nicole's problem. Then Nicole met with Jennifer for a medical evaluation, which included a full gynecological and urological exam. Jennifer checked the internal and external structures, including the clitoris, which is usually omitted during pelvic exams. Through this process she can rule out obvious gynecological problems. Jennifer asked Nicole questions about her present problem, past surgeries, past illnesses, ob-gyn history, family history, and the depression she was being treated for with Paxil. Nicole told Jennifer that she had a

long history of bladder infections, which may also have in-
terfered with her interest in sex since these infections cause
pain and irritation in the urethra.

What followed is the physiologic part of our testing. As
Nicole lay on the examination table, Jennifer inserted a
small flexible pH probe, about the width of a cocktail stirrer,
into Nicole's vagina to measure her vaginal pH. Our nurse-
assistant then recorded a reading of 4.6 on Nicole's chart,
considered in the normal range for a premenopausal woman
(4.5 to 5.1; pH rises in menopausal women who are not on estrogen). After that, Jennifer measured Nicole's clitoral and
labial sensation using a biothesiometer, which is an instru-
ment that detects sensitivity to low- and high-frequency vi-
bration. This provides information about the sensory nerves
to the genital area. Nicole's clitoral and labial sensation were
low. Next, Jennifer inserted a small balloon device into
Nicole's vagina and very slowly inflated it, asking Nicole to
tell her when she felt the first sensation of pressure and then
when it became uncomfortable. This was to measure
Nicole's vaginal compliance, or the ability of the vagina to
relax and lengthen. That was normal.

Finally, Jennifer placed the ultrasound probe, about the
size of a wooden matchstick, against Nicole's clitoris and
labia. The probe allowed Jennifer to see a complete picture
on a television screen of the clitoral and labial anatomy, as
well as the blood flow to Nicole's clitoris, labia, and urethra.
Next, a tampon-sized probe was inserted into her vagina to
measure blood flow to the vagina and uterus. Surprisingly,
given her surgery and what she had told Laura, Nicole had
very good blood flow to all parts of her genital area.

After that, Nicole was given a vibrator and a pair of 3-D

surround sound video glasses. These glasses allow for uninterrupted erotic visual stimulation. Nicole was to watch an erotic video, designed and produced for women, through the glasses and stimulate herself in private with the vibrator for 15 minutes. Before leaving the room, Jennifer told her that the goal was to become maximally aroused so that we could get the best measurements.

After 15 minutes, Jennifer returned and asked Nicole how she was doing. Nicole had not had an orgasm, but shyly said she had enjoyed the vibrator. "I think I need to get one," she said. Jennifer then repeated the three-part exam. Nicole's lubrication and pelvic blood flow had increased significantly poststimulation. Her vaginal elasticity also increased, but her genital sensation did not significantly improve.

After Nicole dressed, we talked with her in our office, where she asked the single most common question in our practice: "Do you think it's in my head?" Laura told her it was absolutely not, but that it was probably her head and body working against each other. Although Nicole did not have any severe anatomic abnormalities, the Paxil she was taking can be associated with sexual function problems. In addition, her previous genital surgery most likely affected the sensory nerves to her labia and minor branches of the clitoris, making it difficult for her to become maximally aroused and have an orgasm. Nicole also had emotional and relationship issues, which in turn made her physical problems worse—a vicious cycle. On an emotional level, the surgery she had had for her vulvar cancer was particularly traumatic. Any woman who faces a life-threatening illness like cancer, particularly in her genital area, is going to feel differently about herself and her body. Nicole seemed to have some negative body image issues from her surgery, which had been mildly disfiguring, and also some fear during sex. Her partner's functioning contributed to her problem.

On Nicole's next visit, she received a single dose of Viagra, the brand name of the drug sildenafil, one hour prior to her evaluation. As we had suspected it might, Nicole's pelvic blood flow tripled poststimulation and her genital sensation increased. She had an orgasm in our clinic, one of her first in years. The Viagra, which increased genital blood flow and sensation, combined with stimulation from the vibrator and the erotic video, seemed to help her overcome the loss of sensation and arousal as a result of her surgery and the SSRI she was taking. She left our clinic with a prescription for Viagra, which she now takes on a regular basis. She was also encouraged to explore the emotional aspect of her problem and was referred to a trained sex therapist in her hometown for further treatment.

Virtually all of our cases at the clinic include some combination of medical, emotional, and relationship problems. It's like a pie chart, but the pieces of the pie are distributed differently. We'll see a woman whose primary problem is medical or physiologic, but because she's experiencing a long-standing problem, it's affecting the way she feels about her body and herself. As a result, her relationship is often in crisis, which makes the physical problems much worse. We've learned that it's very difficult for a woman to separate her sexuality from the context in which she experiences it— that is, in her relationship with her partner. This emphasizes the point that the most important sex organ in the human body is the brain. However, we've learned that physical problems can affect the mind, which in turn affects happiness and sexual satisfaction, and vice versa.

We've had tremendous success using sildenafil for women like Nicole, but it's important to point out that many patients don't even make it to the prescription. Sometimes the diagnosis is a relationship problem, communication difficulties, or a partner who either doesn't know what to do to stimulate her sexually or has sexual function problems of his or her own. We've also learned that even if the problem is purely medical or physiological, medications like it do not always work.

Maria, a 44-year-old medical technician from the Boston suburbs, was a case in point. She came to see us because she had never experienced an orgasm. Attractive, slightly bohemian, and outspoken, Maria had been married for 23 years, with two nearly grown children. She had been raised in Russia, where no one in her family talked about sex, let alone orgasm.

"I knew something was supposed to be happening, and I'd heard the word from reading books, but I knew nothing was happening to me," Maria told Laura. Although Maria had lived in the United States for nearly two decades, no doctor here had been able to help her. She told Laura that when her regular internist had asked her as part of a routine physical about any sexual problems, he had brushed her off when she mentioned that she had never had an orgasm.

"He'd say, 'Oh, all right,' and then go to another question," Maria said.

Ten years earlier, Maria had also seen a psychotherapist about her problems but described the talks with her as too vague to be of help. The psychotherapist had suggested that Maria get a vibrator, but didn't tell her how it worked or what to do with it. At the time, Maria dismissed the vibrator as "stupid." Another therapist had seen Maria and her husband and then just Maria alone, but Maria had become impatient with all the talk and expense and had stopped going. "It was, 'OK, tell me about your fantasies,'" Maria said. "It was interesting for me, but did I really want to pay $100 for this pleasant talk?"

Maria then told Laura that her frustration had led her into an experiment with group sex: she and her husband had made love while another couple, good friends, had sex simultaneously in the same hotel room. "It was so exciting," Maria told Laura. "I loved it." She felt she had came close to orgasm and watched the other woman carefully to see if she could learn what to do. "I was very curious," Maria said. She did in fact learn something, but not what she expected. The other woman, she decided, was faking an orgasm. "I suspect a lot of women don't have orgasms, but just don't talk about it," Maria concluded.

Jennifer put Maria through our standard physical tests, showed her how to use the vibrator, and then left the examination room. When she returned, Maria announced, stunned, that she had just had her first orgasm. "It took me a minute!" Maria said. She was relieved that nothing was wrong with her and amazed that having an orgasm could be so easy.

We never prescribed Viagra for Maria. What she needed was psychosexual education and practical guidance about self-stimulation; she did not have any medical or physical complications and her libido was clearly not the problem. It's also important to point out that Maria's experiments with group sex were not unusual and were in fact symptomatic of her problems. Laura sees a lot of women in long-term relationships who start to question their partners and then reach beyond them to try to figure out what's wrong. They'll often try self-stimulation for the first time, or maybe sex with another partner. Their goal is to rule out a fundamental problem with the partner or the relationship. Often a woman is devastated when she discovers that she has the same sexual problems in an extramarital affair as she does at home with her partner, suggesting to her that the problem is hers rather than her partner's. This experimentation can often put the woman, and sometimes the relationship, into crisis and that is often the point at which she comes to see us.

Since Maria was particularly interested in how a woman climaxes, Laura helped her pick out a vibrator and also advised her about some educational videos (see the Resources section in chapter 9). Maria wanted to learn how to masturbate and felt she needed a visual representation. Laura helped by sketching out the female genitals and pointing out the different components, especially the clitoris. This is something she does for a lot of our patients who grew up being told that self-stimulation is wrong or were never told anything at all.

Maria now checks in regularly with Laura, who suggests practical techniques and devices for her to use at home. Then Maria comes back in and talks about how it all went. Not long ago, Maria told us that she had invited the woman from the group sex experience to her home to watch the video and experiment with the vibrator. Maria said the other woman didn't like the vibrator as much as she did, but Maria still found the experience erotic.

Maria also tried the Eros-CTD, or clitoral therapy device. Developed by UroMetrics, Inc., this is the first intervention to treat female sexual dysfunction approved by the FDA, in May 2000. This device is placed over the clitoris and surrounding tissue and provides gentle suction that the woman controls. It's not meant to replace a vibrator, but it does cause orgasm in some women. Its main purpose is to enhance arousal and to engorge the clitoris and labia by pulling blood into the area. The theory is that, over time, this will prevent fibrosis of the clitoral and labial arteries and the clitoral and labial erectile tissue that typically occurs with aging and menopause. It also increases overall clitoral and labial blood flow. Maria reported that it didn't do much for her, and that she preferred the standard vibrator. But other women, chiefly those who have physiologically based sexual problems, are enthusiastic about it.

Maria now uses the vibrator freely, without shame, embarrassment, or guilt, although not when she has sex with her husband. "We have sex before we go to bed, he falls asleep, I take out my vibrator and do what I have to do, and then I fall asleep," she told Laura. Although Maria and her husband seem to be satisfied with this arrangement for now, we've suggested to her that she and her husband incorporate the vibrator into their foreplay, or perhaps use a smaller, more intense one that can be used during intercourse itself.

Even though Maria could ideally advocate more for herself, at the moment she seems happy. The situation is not affecting her ability to have an orgasm, her sexual satisfaction, or her self-esteem. Our goal is not to tell patients how they should run their sex lives, but to arm them with the information and resources to assume control over their bodies and sexuality. On the other hand, if Maria were to want to change her situation—if she should tell us that she wants her husband to be more responsive, or if she should feel lonely when she stimulates herself after sex—we would start helping her with that. Usually the best course of action in cases like this is couples therapy, but Maria and her partner would both have to be motivated.

One of our most successful cases is that of Paula, a 55-year-old college professor from Boston, married for 22 years. In 1994 she was diagnosed with breast cancer. Over the next three years, Paula had eight breast surgeries and then three pelvic surgeries—the first to remove an ovary, the second for a hysterectomy, and the third to remove pelvic adhesions that developed as a result of the previous two procedures. After the surgeries, Paula was given Paxil for depression.

It was after the hysterectomy that Paula began to notice a decrease in her libido as well as a decrease in her clitoral, labial, and vaginal sensations. Her orgasms, once powerful, became muffled or less intense, but more often didn't occur at all. Paula recovered from the depression and went off the Paxil, but still had almost no desire for sex. "So I began to say to all these caregivers, 'What happened to me?'" Paula told us. "And all of them said, 'Most women your age don't care.' One told me I was only the second woman in 20 years who had cared so much. And this is from women!" The underlying message, Paula said, was "We saved you. What are you complaining about?" She was also convinced that they would never have said those things to a man. Our philosophy is that more women probably care than we think, which is why it is so important that women be made to feel entitled to their sexual response. If not, how will they ever feel comfortable speaking to their doctors about it? It doesn't help when doctors are unable or unwilling to accept and address the problem.

Paula was devastated, then enraged. "I wanted my sexuality back," she said. "I went back to each doctor and said, 'Why didn't you tell me what would happen?'" Paula felt as if she had crashed into a wall. "It really was the first time that ageism and sexism had so profoundly hurt me," she said. "I've had a pretty successful career, and I've been able to manage what life has thrown me, but this just hurt me." In Paula's case, her loss of libido was secondary to the loss of hormones and the fact that sex had been frustrating and unsatisfying. If it isn't enjoyable, why do it?

When Paula came to our office, we saw a self-assured and articulate woman. Unlike other patients, who do not feel entitled to their sexuality, Paula was very firm about what she had lost. She was excited to find us, and adamant about a solution. We also knew that we were the first doctors to take her problem seriously. (Unfortunately, this was no surprise. Laura can't forget a recent comment she saw on the Internet, from a urologist at Harvard, about whether female sexual dysfunction should be included as a subject in a medical study of impotence: "I can't imagine anything more annoying than prompting a parade of unhappy women into urology offices for evaluation of their sexual problems," the doctor wrote. "Do urologists really want to move in this direction? We must be getting desperate for things to keep us occupied professionally.") This is just one blatant example of some physicians' attitudes, which can make it extremely difficult for female patients to talk to their doctors.

When Laura evaluated Paula, she felt there were no significant psychosexual issues at play. Her marriage was stable and she was happy in her relationship. Although her mastectomy and breast reconstruction were enormously difficult experiences, she had worked hard to resolve her body image and emotional issues and trauma from surgery. She seemed to have a medical basis for her problem. Since she was not a candidate for hormonal therapies (estrogen or testosterone) because of her history of breast cancer, and she had experienced enjoyable sex previously, we felt that Paula might benefit from Viagra.

Sure enough, the blood flow to Paula's genital area and her genital sensation increased after she took the medication. She also experienced an orgasm. She was even more successful at home with her husband, and now reports that her libido and 90 percent of her genital sensation are back. Paula discussed the option of topical hormone creams with her gynecologist and oncologist. Due to the type of cancer she had and the lack of recurrence, they both felt that there were some potential options, but that there were still risks associated with them. Paula wanted to restore her sexual response as best she could, and she was willing to take the risk. She received Estring, which is a soft silicone ring impregnated with estrogen that is inserted like a diaphragm into the vagina. It provides a low continuous dose of estrogen to the vaginal tissue to alleviate symptoms of vaginal dryness. (See chapter 5 for a discussion of hormone replacement therapy, estrogen rings, and breast cancer.)

The larger issue was whether there had been damage during her hysterectomy. Our theory is that since we still don't know the precise location of the nerves and blood vessels to the vagina and clitoris that are vital for normal sexual responses, they indeed can be injured during surgery. Although such anatomical ignorance seems astonishing in the twenty-first century, the reality is that we only learned two decades ago where those pelvic nerves and blood vessels are located in men. We have also learned a great deal from rectal surgeons, who have known for years about many of the pelvic nerves and how to avoid them in operations for cancer and colitis in men. For these reasons, one of Jennifer's immediate goals is to determine where these structures are in women and she is currently developing surgeries that will protect and preserve them.

It's important for us to say here that not all women with hysterectomies have complaints of sexual dysfunction. Clearly the surgery doesn't adversely affect all women. One observation of ours is that women who had orgasms with pelvic floor uterine contractions—typically referred to as vaginal or G-spot orgasms—experience the greatest loss when the uterus is removed. Women who, prior to surgery, experienced primarily localized "clitoral orgasms," that is, without pelvic floor and uterine contractions, do not experience the same loss. (We'll get into this in more detail in later chapters, but there are two kinds of orgasms, despite all the myths and misinformation, and one is not better than the other, just different.)

For some women, hysterectomies are necessary, and because they alleviate pain, bleeding, and discomfort, any loss in sensation or of orgasm is offset by relief from the symptoms. One of our patients, a younger woman with endometriosis and bleeding, told us her hysterectomy had improved her sex life because her cramping had finally stopped.

But many other operations women get to "improve" their sexual lives are unnecessary and damaging. Not long ago we had a woman come in with a particularly troubling case. She told us that her boyfriend had grown less responsive and had begun to lose his erection. When she asked why, he told her that "there seems to be a lot of room in there."

She was clearly devastated and embarrassed. Although she was able to reach vaginal orgasm and said she could feel herself "grabbing on" to her boyfriend during intercourse, she went to her gynecologist and told him, "My boyfriend says I'm too loose." The doctor then said he could give her an operation to tighten her up. Since we didn't see the woman before the surgery, we have no idea of the extent of her problem, or even if it was a problem at all. It is quite possible that the problem may have been with her boyfriend. Some women, however, are born with or develop weak supporting tissues in their pelvis, which become more pronounced as they grow older. In healthy women, aging, vaginal childbirths, and prolonged labors are the primary causes of pelvic support problems, which may potentially cause damage to the muscles in the pelvic floor and result in the perception of a "looser" vagina. (See chapter 4 for more information about pelvic floor disorders.)

The doctor ended up performing a version of the operation for women with vaginal prolapse, or lifting and tightening the vaginal wall. We do not know for sure if she indeed had vaginal prolapse (loosening and falling of the vagina). After her recovery, she found that her lubrication remained the same, and that she was able to have clitoral orgasms. But she told us that she no longer had sensation in her vagina and was unable to have vaginal orgasms.

It is frustrating to see so many women who have been persuaded to have unnecessary surgeries to enhance their genital appearance and then lose their sexual function as a result. Unfortunately, we think this is a reflection of not only the negative way in which women view their genitals in general, but also the fact that what is considered "attractive" is determined by men.

．　　　．　　　．

When we're not in our clinic, Laura sees patients for ongoing therapy and handles our administrative work. Jennifer is either performing surgery on women with urologic problems or is in the lab, studying vaginal and clitoral muscle physiology and performing cadaver dissections to better understand female pelvic anatomy. For the muscle physiology experiments, tissue samples are held in place with clips and stretched in a large tube called an organ chamber. Jennifer then tests the effects of different drugs and hormones on the tissues. She is also able to stimulate the nerves in the tissues and then evaluate how the tissues react with or without certain drugs. She is also looking at the effects of a new drug that increases mucus production in the cervix, which increases vaginal lubrication.

The goal of her research is to help develop new medications for women and to understand the female sexual response. Jennifer discovered that several medications and hormones enhance sexual responses in female animals. This information is being used to tailor drug development and future clinical trials in women. She also discovered that vaginal tissue responds differently, depending on whether it is in the upper or lower vagina. This suggests that drugs may have different effects depending on where in the vagina they are placed and on the inherent structure of the tissue. Her research is ongoing, and we are optimistic about future findings.

In 1998 and 1999, we evaluated the physiological sexual responses of 48 women pre- and post-Viagra, then followed up with a questionnaire after the women had taken Viagra for six weeks at home. The results: 67 percent said their ability to have an orgasm increased after taking it. More than 70 percent said they felt more sensation in the genital area during intercourse, sexual stimulation, or foreplay.

We should note that other studies have determined that Viagra had little effect on female sexual dysfunction, including the first placebo-controlled sildenafil study, led by Dr. Rosemary Basson of Vancouver General Hospital. That study found that the drug did no better than a placebo among 577 women. But our study was different in that Laura carefully screened patients beforehand, eliminating those with emotional and relationship problems that would be better addressed by therapy. We excluded women who had primary complaints of hypoactive sexual desire disorder—that is, women with a longtime lack of interest in sex, which is often emotionally based. In addition, all the women we selected had to already have adequate levels of testosterone, the "hormone of desire," either naturally or through replacement, in order to be included in the study. We also excluded women with a history of sexual abuse, major depression, or a psychiatric disorder that required medication. We did include women who were taking selective seratonin reuptake inhibitors (SSRIs) like Prozac and Zoloft for depression, provided that the women had been free of anxiety or depression for at least a year. Most important, we selected patients who had previously enjoyed sex.

To be evaluated, a woman had to exhibit symptoms of sexual arousal disorder. That is, she could not attain or maintain adequate genital lubrication or swelling during sex and to have a decreased sensation in her clitoris, vagina, or labia—problems that are often medically based. She also had to have been in a satisfying relationship for at least the past six months, be comfortable with self-stimulation, and be satisfied with her partner's ability to sexually stimulate her.

Our goal with these requirements was to narrow down the pool of women to those who appeared to have physiological problems; we already knew from our experience with our patients that Viagra is of limited use for psychological or relationship problems. Half of the participants were menopausal, and almost a third had had hysterectomies.

We found that Viagra significantly increased the blood flow to the vagina, clitoris, labia, and urethra in all 48 women. Seventy percent of the women also reported that their overall sexual experience had significantly improved.

The positive findings of these initial evaluations led to a larger scale study that is currently under way. If this study shows a positive effect, suggesting a role for Viagra in the treatment of women with sexual dysfunction, FDA approval may not be far off.

CHAPTER TWO

The History of Female Sexuality

Why does the field of women's sexual health lag 20 to 30 years behind that of men? Why haven't women received the same attention? To understand the present, we have to consider the past. Although a comprehensive history of female sexuality is beyond our scope in this book, we think a brief overview—chiefly of what was happening in Europe and in nineteenth- and twentieth-century America—will explain how so many women came to be the second-class sexual citizens they are today.

Little is known definitively about sexual behavior in ancient times, and it's questionable how much relevance the sexual practices of the people of Mesopotamia have to our own, but a few things bear mentioning. From the time of the earliest recorded history, about 3000 B.C., women were considered property, valued for reproduction. Adultery was not a sin of morality, but a crime of trespass against a husband. In ancient Greece, where a woman had no more political or legal rights than a slave, she was simply called *gyne*, which meant "bearer of children." Her womb defined her. Plato, in fact, was one of the first in a long line of misinformed men throughout history to decree that an inactive uterus was a cause of hysteria, a women's disease that caused nervousness, fainting spells, and insomnia. As he wrote in his dialogue *Timaeus*, the womb was an "indwelling creature desirous of childbearing" that if left "barren too long after puberty" would begin to wander around the body, cut off respiration and cause in its sufferer "extreme anguish"—an apparent reference to menstruation and menstrual cramps.

By the second century A.D., the medical writer Galen described hysteria as a uterine disease that was caused by sexual deprivation. He recommended intercourse or mastur-bation as cures. The disease, after all, had the classic symp-toms of chronic sexual arousal: anxiety, irritability, erotic fantasy, sensations of heaviness in the abdomen. Galen also said that passionate women were at particular risk for the disease.

If the Greeks viewed women as chattel and the Romans considered infertility as grounds for divorce, the Christian church that moved into the political void after the fall of Rome went even further. The church fathers deemed sex un-savory and women a threat to male salvation. One of the most influential of the church thinkers was St. Augustine, who had once lived with a mistress and had had a hard time controlling his own lust. After joining the church, he became guilt-ridden and disgusted by his sexual desires, renounced them, adopted a life of celibacy, and imposed his ideas on everyone else. He also wrote that he knew nothing that brought "the manly mind down from the heights more than a woman's caresses and that joining of bodies." Procreation with such "temptresses" was to be accomplished by passion-less, purposeful intercourse. At a time of widespread illiter-acy, when reading and writing were the preserve of the church, his conclusions were accepted, propagated by word of mouth, and became, over time, absolute.

Although Asian attitudes were far freer—the *Kama Sutra* of India, compiled sometime between the third and fifth centuries, is a detailed sex manual glorifying sexual pleasure for both men and women—the early Christian traditions set the tone over the next centuries in the West. The chastity belt of the Middle Ages was a torturous device constructed on a metal frame that stretched between a woman's legs from front to back. It had two small openings for urination and defecation but prevented penetration. Most important, it gave husbands the power to lock up their wives (their sexual property) as they would their money.

The rebirth of the arts and humanism during the Renaissance freed some sexual attitudes, as did the sixteenth-century Protestant Reformation, led by Martin Luther and John Calvin. In their rebellion against the Pope, the reformers concluded that sex within marriage was permissible not only for procreation, but also "to lighten and ease the cares and sadnesses of household affairs, or to endear each other"—a revolution of sorts.

The Puritans who migrated from England to America brought with them the attitudes of the Protestant Reformation, and so placed a new importance on sex within marriage. But as anyone who has ever read *The Scarlet Letter* knows, they went to extremes on sexual transgression outside marriage. It was a harsh new world, requiring much personal discipline. Perhaps they felt challenged by such "savage" practices of the Native Americans as premarital sex, polygamy, and homosexuality. (However, Hope Ashby, a therapist and cross-cultural sexuality expert, says that after the settlers began raping Indian women, it was the Native Americans who finally enacted laws prohibiting such violent behavior.) The Puritan clergy preached that man (but especially woman) was as full of sin, as one minister put it, "as a toad is of poi-son." The community had to take charge of the weak-of-faith, which was potentially everyone. Those giving in to adultery, if found, were flogged, put in stocks, or forced to make public confessions. Men, naturally, were considered more rational and able to control their passions than women, who were chastised by ministers for dressing improperly and luring men into sin. Sexual crimes, of course, involved two people, usually a man and a woman, but women were more often prosecuted and convicted.

By the nineteenth century, virtuous women of the middle class were expected to embrace modesty, personify purity, and lack all sexual desire. The Victorian era in America transformed the middle-class housewife into no less than a guardian of the public morality. Her place was at home with her children, on a pedestal of innocence, protecting the fam-ily's decency and social position. She endured sex with her husband for procreation, but if her husband was a decent soul he subjected her to his animal urges as infrequently as possible. As puzzling as it seems now, many middle-class women readily accepted the view that they were without sexual passion, whether from the social pressures of a self-conscious middle class, or ignorance, or both.

At the same time, "hysteria" was apparently pandemic. If the disease was in fact chronic sexual frustration, as Rachel P. Maines argues in her book *The Technology of Orgasm,* an en-tertaining but serious history of the vibrator, women sought relief through one of the few acceptable outlets: going to the doctor's office and being massaged to orgasm. Maines writes that Western doctors performed the "routine chore" of re-lieving hysterical patients' symptoms with manual genital massage until a woman reached orgasm, or, as it was known under clinical conditions, the "hysterical paroxysm." The vibrator, invented by a British physician in the 1880s, was a direct response to doctors who wanted help performing this procedure.

There is also evidence that not all nineteenth-century middle-class women were as Victorian behind closed doors as in public. The cultural historian Peter Gay, for example, has quoted extensively in his work from the diary of Mabel Loomis Todd, a proper New England wife who had a decadelong extramarital affair with Austin Dickinson, Emily Dickinson's brother. But Mabel Todd also reveled in the eroticism of her marriage to her husband, David Todd: "We retired at seven and had a magnificient evening, David and I," Mabel Todd wrote in her diary in February 1882. "I shall never forget it, so I'll not write about it." The entry was followed by two symbols indicating the couple had intercourse twice that night. Three years earlier, while on vacation in New York's Finger Lakes, she wrote that they "went in the steamer Schuyler from Geneva to Watkins, on the beautiful Seneca Lake—oh! How we loved each other! And what a glorious and beautiful evidence of it we had in our room, before dinner, at the Glen Mountain House!"

But Mabel Todd was probably the exception. Most Victorian women repressed their sexuality to such a degree that most men and some women viewed prostitution as a necessary evil that allowed the male a natural outlet for his lust. The nineteenth century was a time when prostitution readily flourished as the rise of cities and the expanding frontier—with men out on their own, and wives and families left behind—brought sexuality into the marketplace. In some silver-mining towns in Nevada, prostitution was the largest occupational category for women other than housewife. By the time of the American Civil War, a guidebook of fashionable brothels listed 106 establishments in New York City and 57 in Philadelphia.

Rampant prostitution in turn provoked the first sexual reform movement, which began among the white women of a rising commercial class (and a few freed slaves) in Boston and upstate New York and was part of the larger social reform movement—against intemperance, poverty, and slavery—of the 1830s. To middle-class white women reformers, prostitution was a threat to public morality but also to the health of husbands at a time of cholera and spreading syphilis. And since many prostitutes were women of color, white women were less than happy that their husbands were being serviced by "colored people." Unfortunately for the reformers, most prostitutes didn't think they needed reforming and generally resisted efforts to take up sewing or become household servants. For women of color, who had a lower overall social status, prostitution afforded them a better income, not to mention a moderate level of power.

After the Civil War, a broader movement led by women launched an attack on prostitution. The movement included supporters like the suffragists Susan B. Anthony and Elizabeth Cady Stanton, who argued that the same standard of morality should apply to both sexes. In 1867 they blocked a move to legalize prostitution in New York State. By the turn of the century, this "social purity" movement had not ended prostitution but evidently had had its effect on middle-class marriage, as two remarkable sex surveys of the era show. As is common for this era, racism and discrimination precluded women of color from participating in these surveys.

Katharine B. Davis, a Vassar-educated settlement-house

worker and later the superintendent of a women's prison, conducted a survey of 2,200 women, most of them born before 1890, and found that the majority described sex as of limited importance in their married lives, just as the social purity reformers preached. Clelia D. Mosher, a doctor and college professor who surveyed 45 of her women patients, had similar results. Even those women who liked sex—and in the Mosher survey, a third said they usually experienced orgasm—were filled with guilt and confusion. One woman, for example, listed pleasure among the purposes of sex, but qualified herself by writing, "but not necessarily a legitimate one." Half of the women in the Mosher survey and 40 percent in the Davis survey said they didn't have enough instruction about sex before marriage. Interestingly, three-fourths of the women in the Davis study practiced some form of contraception. Rhythm and withdrawal were the most common methods of the era, but couples also used condoms, vaginal sponges, and the diaphragm, which had been patented in 1846 under the title The Wife's Protector.

By early in the next century, Sigmund Freud was questioning almost every aspect of sex as it had been previously understood. Freud, a Viennese neurologist and the founder of psychoanalysis, concluded that sex was a primary force in human life. He also created a theory of psychosexual development that began in earliest childhood. In his most famous formulation, the Oedipus complex, Freud stated that a young boy is inevitably sexually attracted to his mother but also has castration anxiety, or an unconscious fear that his father will punish him by removing his penis. Freud's ideas were revolutionary and had enormous impact on attitudes in America in that they promoted indulging rather than suppressing sexual desire. In more recent decades, Freud has been attacked by feminists and other critics for his phallocentricism and his misunderstanding of female sexuality.

Freud believed that young girls suffer from both penis envy and an Electra complex, or a desire to sexually possess their fathers and replace their mothers, whom they blame for their deficient bodies. Freud also viewed the clitoris as a kind of inferior penis, which girls would naturally discover and manipulate during self-exploration. But as a girl grew up, Freud said, she should abandon her childish interest in her clitoris and focus on the vagina, the receptive organ for the penis. In a telling affirmation of such attitudes, one woman reported to us that her obstetrician told her apologetically after delivering her daughter (instead of the son she suspected from the ultrasound), "Well, your baby doesn't have a penis, but has a nice place to put one." In a view that still permeates our culture, Freud decreed that clitoral orgasms were immature but that vaginal orgasms were "authentic."

Writing at the same time as Freud was Havelock Ellis, an English doctor who is less well known today but who had a far more positive impact on women's attitudes toward their sexuality. Ellis, a romantic who is sometimes called the prophet of modern sexuality, wrote the six-volume *Studies in the Psychology of Sex*, a widely read banquet of the varieties of sexual expression. He believed in female eroticism and the need of women to fulfill their strong sexual needs. He also argued that the emphasis on sex as a means of reproduction was a repressive influence on female sexuality. Freud, he once said, was "an extravagant genius—the greatest figure in psychology, who was almost always wrong."

Ellis's ideas took deep root among small groups of American radicals based in New York City, chiefly Greenwich

Village, who experimented with sex and believed in a new, emancipated woman who had the same passions as men. Their ideas were a long way from the "social purity" crusades, and helped lead to a new politics of sexuality, the battle over birth control. In 1916 Margaret Sanger, a mother of three from the suburbs of New York—and at one point a lover of Havelock Ellis, according to Sanger's biographer, Ellen Chesler—opened a birth control clinic in a working-class neighborhood of Brooklyn, where she was arrested and jailed for providing contraceptive information without a doctor's presence. Her subsequent trial gave the birth control movement its best publicity ever. Above all, birth control—that is, the use of contraceptive devices like the diaphragm that Sanger advocated, rather than abstinence, rhythm, or withdrawal—reflected a seismic shift in the sexual norms of the middle class. Promoting contraception over abstinence reflected an indisputable acceptance of women having sex for the sole purpose of enjoyment.

By the middle of the century, a little-known professor of zoology at Indiana University was able to show how much private sexual behavior differed from publicly acceptable norms. He was Alfred Kinsey, who in 1948 published a cultural milestone, *Sexual Behavior in the Human Male. Sexual Behavior in the Human Female* appeared five years later. The studies, based on face-to-face interviews with 12,000 people, were written in textbook prose that described more exhaustively than ever before the sexual habits of ordinary Americans (but only white Americans). In exacting detail, Kinsey tabulated the frequency of masturbation, premarital and marital intercourse, extramarital sex, and homosexuality.

The findings, at least to traditionalists, were shocking. The study of the men showed that nearly 90 percent had had premarital intercourse and half had engaged in extramarital sex. Kinsey also reported that more than a third of adult males had had a homosexual experience to the point of orgasm, while 4 percent said they were exclusively homosexual as adults.

As startling as these results were to heterosexuals in the late 1940s, it was the survey of women that ignited the furor. Even then, few Americans were ready to hear that women were as capable of orgasm as men. Newspapers, community leaders, and educators fell over themselves to condemn the book as amoral. But those willing to ignore the denunciations, and many were, found that the data showed something striking: "a distinct and steady increase in the number of females reaching orgasm in their marital coitus." Kinsey's results showed that more of the older women interviewed never reached orgasm during intercourse but that more of the younger women almost always did. (Older women were those born in the late nineteenth century and younger women were those born in the 1920s.) Kinsey cited the freer attitudes of society and the more extensive premarital sexual experiences of women as among the reasons for the change.

Thirteen years later, in 1966, William H. Masters and Virginia E. Johnson, a physician and a behavioral scientist at Washington University Medical School in St. Louis, became internationally known with the publication of *Human Sexual Response*. The book, which described their work observing and recording human sexual activity at their laboratory in St. Louis, for the first time clarified and described the female sexual response as consisting of four phases: excitement, plateau, orgasm, and resolution.

The excitement phase, Masters and Johnson said, is marked by vaginal lubrication, vaginal and clitoral swelling, and quickness of breath. In the plateau phase, increased blood flow to the genitals causes the tissues in the lower third of the vagina to swell, narrowing the vaginal opening by at least 30 percent and ensuring that the outer vagina will in effect grip the penis upon insertion. The inner lips of the vagina also double or even triple in thickness, which pushes the outer lips apart. The orgasm stage occurs when stimulation of the clitoris or pressure on the vaginal wall or cervix causes body tension and pelvic engorgement to build to a climax. Rhythmic, involuntary, and pleasurable muscular contractions of the uterus, the outer third of the vagina and the anal sphincter expel blood and tension from the pelvic tissues. The resolution phase is the return to the nonaroused state, when the physiological changes reverse.

Masters and Johnson also said that all orgasms in women are clitoral, a pronouncement that still causes confusion today. Anne Koedt, in her classic 1969 essay, "The Myth of the Vaginal Orgasm," said that "the sexually mature female who reached orgasm through vaginal penetration was the creation of male sexual preferences." (There are in fact different types of orgasms, which we address in chapter 3.)

The 1960s brought some of the most sweeping social changes of the century, and much of it directly affected female sexuality—not all for the good. In the first year of the decade, the Food and Drug Administration approved the use of female oral contraceptives, giving women direct control over their own fertility. The pill severed sex from reproduction in a way that earlier barrier methods never had. No longer did a woman have to interrupt lovemaking to insert a diaphragm, and no longer did she have to negotiate with her lover to use a condom. But although the pill ushered in an authentic revolution, giving a woman the freedom to have sex when she wanted and with whom she wanted, it also put a new burden on her to be sexually "liberated." Women in the nineteenth century had suffered because they weren't supposed to enjoy sex or were married to men who didn't care if they didn't. Women of the twentieth century had the new pressures of being drawn into sex much earlier in a relationship, with expectations from men that they should be sexual adventurers or at least multiorgasmic. "Placed on the defensive, they were rapidly losing the right to say no that nineteenth-century feminists had struggled to obtain," write John D'Emilio and Estelle B. Freedman in *Intimate Matters: A History of Sexuality in America.*

Similarly, the rebellions of the 1960s—against the Vietnam War, racial inequality, poverty, American materialism, and traditional notions of sexual morality—did not necessarily mean that women were beneficiaries. In fact, women of the sixties' protest movements were often sexually exploited and regularly denigrated by the male leaders, which in part led them out of frustration and anger to break away and form their own movement centered on "women's liberation." When Shulamith Firestone, one of the early organizers of the feminist movement, spoke at a 1969 rally of radical groups about women's oppression, she faced cries from the men of "take her off the stage and fuck her!" Male antidraft organizers even popularized the slogan "Girls say yes to guys who say no."

The sexual revolution was a largely Western phenomenon. It did not have the same impact in Asia, except among some of the affluent and educated classes. Even so, any increased sexual activity among women did not necessarily lead to increased sexual satisfaction. In India in the mid-1980s, for example, a survey of 695 middle-class women by a Bombay sex therapist, R. H. Dastur, found that only 10 to 15 percent reached orgasm during intercourse. Dastur, the author of *Sex Power: The Conquest of Sexual Inadequacy,* found that the rest "merely submitted to sex and went through it mechanically with the idea that it was their duty in order to have a male child." The Indian psychoanalyst Sudhir Kakar, in a 1987 lecture delivered at the University of California at Berkeley, spoke of the "widespread sexual misery" among all classes in India.

In other parts of Asia, such as Japan, sexual pleasure has been largely the province of men, and in many cases separate from marriage. Wives and mothers have always been honored as the essential nurturers of the next generation of Japanese, but their own sexual needs have often been an afterthought. It is not that women are ignorant of the sexual arts: prostitutes, bar hostesses, and some of the traditional geishas of old are well known to have been skilled in giving and receiving pleasure. But for the average woman in Japan, sex has traditionally been seen as more of a family obligation than a focus of sharing and intimacy.

In the 1980s in the United States, two forces—AIDS and a modern "purity" movement under the guise of "family values"—caused a retrenchment against American society's openness toward sex. AIDS in particular continues to affect attitudes. Even though more people than ever are living full, long lives with HIV and AIDS-related illnesses, negative social judgments and fear about how the disease is transmitted have expanded to a larger social judgment about sexuality in general. Sex will always be seen in our time as joyous and life-enhancing, but AIDS has added a dimension of fear and possible death. Hepatitis, especially hepatitis C, has had some of the same effect.

Four decades after the freedom provided by the birth control pill, couples must use condoms again. They also have to ask about and know their partner's sexual history. Sexually active women need to be tested for HIV and other sexually transmitted diseases that have surfaced in recent decades, especially herpes, chlamydia, and human papilloma virus (HPV), which is related to cervical and anal cancer. Recent studies have implied that many teenage girls are afraid of sex, and that fewer have intercourse than did girls 15 or 20 years ago. But most of our patients, who are in their twenties and older, generally know about HIV prevention and are not as frightened as people were at the beginning of the epidemic. That may be because the specter of AIDS has become incorporated into the way we experience our sexuality, or at least the way single people experience it.

Other social forces are more subtle. We've found that many women are still influenced by the social taboo that nice girls shouldn't feel entitled to their own sexual satisfaction. Many of our patients worry that their male partners will be intimidated or threatened or made to feel inadequate if they advocate for what they want sexually. Many know that they're supposed to be sexual, but it's a bigger step for a woman to feel so entitled to sexual satisfaction that she asks her partner for what she wants or "coaches" him on what to do to please her—or actually goes to a doctor's office to attend to a sexual problem. That's placing a tremendous amount of importance on that part of her life. Women of all ages, professions, and backgrounds still fear that advocating for their sexuality is wrong and doing so would damage their status as "nice girls."

Women of color have faced a specific sexual social challenge. Years ago they were placed into two categories: either a "Jezebel" or a "Lolita," an insatiable woman always ready and wanting sex, or a "mammy" or an "Aunt Jemima," a woman who had no sexual persona at all. Hope Ashby says that the racism of the American South supported this notion of black women as loose or nymphomaniacal. The stereotypes are still pervasive today and have a profound impact on how sexuality is experienced among this population of women.

Patients will often tell us, "You know, I feel awkward talking about this, or maybe I'm just crazy to think this is so important." Younger women may know that it's important, but often they're still not really comfortable talking to their partners about sex. A younger woman is still worried, for instance, that her partner might feel inadequate if she's not having an orgasm, or worse, that he'll leave her if he finds out. Even the most liberated women still fake orgasms.

And yet we are optimistic and excited about new attitudes and the new millennium. We tend to forget how much sexuality has become part of our everyday lives. Society's growing openness about sex in the last few decades— reflected in the publication of books as diverse as Helen Gurley Brown's *Sex and the Single Girl*, Alex Comfort's *Joy of Sex*, and the feminist health and sex manual *Our Bodies, Ourselves*—have made many women more comfortable with their own sexuality. We've also seen how the widespread use of sildenafil has led people to talk more openly about sexual problems. When Bob Dole discussed erectile dysfunction—

his own, in particular—on national television, that opened doors and brought men as well as women "out of the closet" with their sexual function complaints. The fact that these discussions are occurring in our homes and in our offices is exciting and means that the lines of communication are now open.

CHAPTER THREE

Female Sexual Anatomy and Response

Gail is an attractive 23-year-old, with a cheerful, open disposition and a recent history of dyspareunia, or vaginal pain during sexual intercourse. Her initial symptoms were burning sensations in her vagina after sex, but by the time she came to see us, intercourse with her husband had become so painful—she said it felt as if he was wearing sandpaper on his penis—that she had long given up on any physical intimacy.

Gail, a computer processor from Columbus, Ohio, also told us that before the dyspareunia started, she had never had an orgasm, either alone or with her husband. They had been married for two years. "He would have the orgasm, and I just felt, 'Oh, that's OK, mine will come in time,'" Gail said. "So I watched, and waited, and it never did."

Gail had a history of recurrent urinary tract infections, and it seemed as if her problems were a mix of physiological complaints combined with her very understandable fear of pain. However, the first hurdle we needed to address was her lack of knowledge about her body, in particular her sexual anatomy. We discovered that she had no idea what an orgasm was, what pleased her, or how to masturbate. "I'm just clueless about my body," she admitted. Not surprisingly, she told us that her family, while very nurturing and loving, was also very strict and conservative about sexuality and had never given her any information about sex in general. This is not an unusual history. Many children have been raised into maturity guided only by a book offered by the parents, by tangential references to procreation-oriented sexuality, or by the experiences of acquaintances. "My parents never sat us down and said the word 'sex' in our house," Gail told Laura. "I just picked up things from TV." She said she recalled seeing her parents kiss each other only twice in her life. The message, she said, was clear: sex was dirty, and perhaps even wrong.

After Gail met with Laura, Jennifer began the medical evaluation. When she inserted even the small probe into Gail's vagina, Gail became extremely uncomfortable. She was physically healthy, although she did have thinning of her vaginal lining. We suggested that she use the vibrator, by holding it lightly over her clitoris. To her amazement, it didn't take her long to have an orgasm alone in our examination room. She was also a bit embarrassed. "It just made me feel so bad and so dirty," she said. We had to explain to her that her orgasm was a normal, healthy response. She had no pain during the clitoral stimulation, which was a breakthrough for her.

We prescribed estrogen cream to help increase lubrication and improve the lining of her vagina. We also prescribed testosterone cream to help enhance sensation and to improve her inner labia. She was given a list of resources to learn more about her sexuality, sexual anatomy, and self-stimulation. We sat down with her and went over a catalog of sex toys and aids and then helped her pick out her own vibrator, which she sent away for. Until Gail learned how to stimulate herself, it was unlikely that anyone else would be able to do it for her. She would then need to feel comfortable enough to teach her partner how to stimulate her. There is still a widely held myth that a man is supposed to know exactly what to do to sexually satisfy his partner. Unfortunately, men are rarely provided with any formal sex education beyond what they learn from often misinformed friends or erotic films that are, with few exceptions, typically geared toward a male's sexual pleasure, not a female's. The reality is that most men need and actually want to learn from partners who are not embarrassed to guide and teach them about women's sexual needs. It is therefore no surprise that many people, including physicians, lack fundamental understanding of the nuances of women's sexual response. Courses in human sexuality for physicians will help doctors learn how to effectively treat women with sexual function complaints and how to teach their patients to feel comfortable talking about sexual topics.

We're still working with Gail on the dyspareunia, which we believe is due to vulvadynia or vestibulitis, a nonspecific inflammation and irritation of the inner labia and vaginal opening that causes pain. (See chapter 4 for a more detailed explanation.) Her condition has improved but is still not completely cured. Because of the association of her vaginal symptoms with urinary symptoms of frequency, urgency, and pain, we are helping her change her diet. We have found that certain foods, such as chocolate, citrus fruits, nuts, and alcoholic beverages, can exacerbate both the urinary as well as vaginal symptoms in women with vulvadynia.

Gail is now working at changing her negative attitudes

toward sexuality and sexual expression and is using the vibrator alone. She is now able to have orgasms. Although she is still struggling with some pain, she feels better about her body and her sexuality and is delighted that she is now able to achieve orgasm. The next step is to incorporate her husband in the stimulation phase, and from there open up the lines of communication and work toward a broader, more satisfying sexual relationship. As more research is done in the field and new information and treatments become available for vulvadynia and vestibulitis, we will continue to adjust Gail's medication and therapy.

By far the most important thing we did for Gail was to provide her with basic information and the permission, in essence, to explore her own body. Although many of our patients are comfortable with masturbation, others have absorbed the message still prevalent in our culture that the female genitals are unattractive and a part of the female body that a woman herself shouldn't touch. We're a long way from some cultures in the developing world, where women are sent from their homes during their menstrual periods to avoid the supposed contamination of food, but we're still a society that uses feminine hygiene products to mask the "odor" of the vagina. Some of our patients continue to douche or use genital deodorants, which we strongly discourage because they so often cause dryness, irritation, or itching. They can also increase the potential for infection.

Furthermore, genital cosmetic surgery in which lasers and other surgical techniques are used to even out the labia, tighten the vaginal opening, and make women's genitals look younger and redder should be avoided. Such surgery has the potential for doing more damage than good by injuring the nerves and blood supply to the labia and vagina, as well as the vaginal muscle and cells lining the vaginal canal. Women should never be made to feel embarrassed or self-conscious about their bodies. There are too many preconceived norms, established primarily by men, about what makes female genitalia attractive. One of our patients is now trying to undo the work of a surgeon who so radically reconstructed and tightened her vagina, supposedly to make her genitals more attractive to her husband and to give him more pleasure during intercourse, that she ended up with genital pain and even less sensitivity than before. We have to believe that if women were conditioned to feel more positive about their bodies in general, these radical interventions wouldn't be happening.

Many of our patients who are at ease with masturbation and touching themselves have still never taken a close look at their own genitals. Since understanding our sexual anatomy is a first step toward pleasure, we offer here brief but important descriptions of a woman's sexual organs. We'll also describe the role of the breasts, anus, rectum, and buttocks in sexual stimulation, how sexual arousal and orgasm occur, and the difference between clitoral and pelvic floor orgasms.

External Organs

Genitals: The sexual organs in the pelvic region of both women and men are called the genitals. In women the genitals consist of both external sex organs, collectively called the vulva, and the internal organs, which include the vagina, uterus, fallopian tubes, and ovaries. In men the external genitals consist of the penis, scrotum, and testes. The internal genital structures involved in the transmission of sperm and seminal fluid in men include the vas deferens, seminal vesicles, epididymis, and prostate.

Vulva: We've found that many people confuse the vagina and vulva. Others have never heard of the word. The vulva is the entire outer visible genital area, including the mons pubis, the labia, the clitoris, the perineum, the urethra, and the anus (see figure 3.1). Pubic hair runs down the length of the vulva, sometimes reaching as far as the upper thighs. A woman can have a lot of pubic hair or a little. The first wisps of pubic hair appear at puberty, grow steadily as a woman matures, and thin out after menopause.

Figure 3.1 External sex organs (vulva)

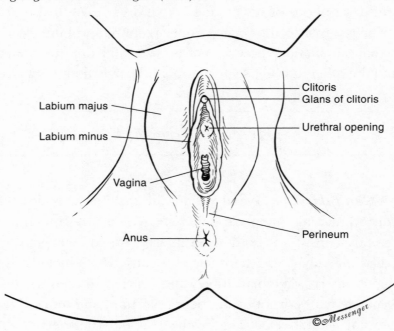

Mons pubis* or *mons veneris: Latin for mound of Venus, the Roman goddess of love. The mons pubis, or mons, is the fatty mound of flesh covered by pubic hair that is directly over the pubic bone. The area has a number of nerve endings, and many women find that stimulation of the mons, or direct pressure, can lead to sexual arousal.

Labia: Composed of the outer lips (labia majora) and inner lips (labia minora). The anatomic counterpart of the scrotum in men, the labia are the fleshy flaps of skin that fold together over the opening of the vagina. Pubic hair grows on the outer lips, while the inner lips are smooth and rich in small blood vessels. Both have many sensory nerve endings and are an important source of sexual stimulation. When a woman is aroused, the labia darken, become engorged with blood, and move apart, opening the way to the vagina. Changes also occur in color, size, and texture of the labia with aging and menopause. Menopausal women who are not taking hormone replacement therapy, as well as pre- and perimenopausal women with low testosterone levels, often have thinning and shrinkage of the inner and outer labia. Sometimes the labia minora actually become so atrophied that they fuse with the labia majora, making them almost indistinguishable. Dryness, irritation, and pain can occur as a result. (See the HRT section in chapter 5 for more information.)

Clitoris: The clitoris is the most sensitive area of a woman's genitals (see figure 3.2), and is composed of the same tissue as the most sensitive part of a man's penis, the glans. Stimulating the clitoris either manually or orally causes many women to reach intense orgasms. Most of it, however, is not visible, which is one reason its size is still such a matter of debate. What you can see if you sit with your legs spread in front of a small hand-held mirror is its head, or the clitoral glans. The glans is the tiny knob of flesh, about the size of a pea, right below the mons, where the inner lips join to form a soft fold of skin, or clitoral hood. If you gently push up the hood, you should be able to see the clitoral glans.

Although most medical textbooks still label the glans as "the clitoris," the actual clitoris is far more extensive. In 1981 the Federation of Feminist Women's Health Centers redefined the clitoris in its book, *A New View of a Woman's Body*, as a structure that includes not only the hood and glans but also a shaft, legs, muscles, and bulbs. In 1998 an Australian urologist, Helen O'Connell, described the glans as attached to a shaft of pyramid-shaped erectile tissue about the size of the first joint of the thumb. O'Connell based her findings on the dissections of cadavers and the use of 3-D photography techniques. She also described the many nerves, blood vessels, and smooth muscles of the clitoris, which is made of the same erectile tissue as the penis and which swells during arousal. (See figure 5.1.)

To find the body of the clitoris, which together with the glans is two to four centimeters long, you need to feel directly behind the glans to the shaft, which feels like a firm, movable cord right under the skin. Attached to the shaft are the two clitoral legs that you can't see or feel at all. The legs, or crura, are nine to eleven centimeters long, and flair backward into the body, spreading out like a wide wishbone; they attach to the inferior aspect of the pubic bone. The clitoral bulbs—usually called the bulbs of the vestibule and rarely recognized in medical textbooks as part of the clitoris—are two bundles of erectile tissue that extend down the sides of the

Figure 3.2 The clitoris

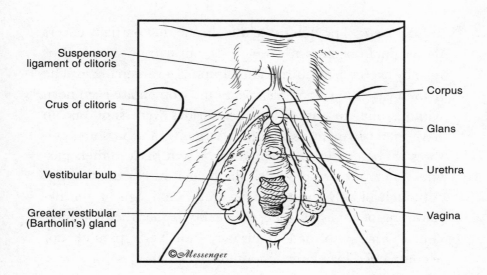

Suspensory
ligament of clitoris

Crus of clitoris

Vestibular bulb

Greater vestibular
(Bartholin's) gland

Corpus

Glans

Urethra

Vagina

©*Messenger*

vestibule, the area just outside the vagina, and surround the urethra. The vestibular bulbs are connected to the glans of the clitoris.

During sexual arousal, the bulbs, legs, shaft, and glans of the clitoris become firm and filled with blood. The legs and the bulbs are both surrounded by muscle tissue (the bulbo-cavernosus and ischiocavernosus muscles), which, when contracted, help to create tension during arousal and the spasms felt during orgasm.

Perineum: The hairless area of skin between the bottom of the labia and the anus, which is sometimes torn or intentionally cut during childbirth, in what is called an episiotomy, to allow for the head of the baby to pass through the vaginal opening. Like other parts of the genitals, the perineum contains sensory nerve endings and is sensitive to the touch. It can be a source of arousal in some women.

Hymen: The thin tissue membrane that partially covers the vaginal opening in young girls, but can be stretched or torn by exercise, masturbation, tampons, or intercourse. The hymen varies in size and shape. Some women are even born without one. In earlier societies, brides were supposed to have intact hymens as proof of virginity, and in some cultures women with torn hymens were sent back to their parents. Intercourse may stretch the hymen rather than tear it. Although bloody sheets were a traditional sign of the deflowering of a virgin bride, the reality is that the first intercourse for a woman is usually not very painful nor accompanied by a large amount of bleeding.

Internal Organs

Vagina: The vagina is shaped like a tube, usually around five to seven inches long, and tilts upward and posteriorly toward the small of your back (see figure 3.3). Usually the walls of the vagina gently touch each other, but during childbirth the vagina has the amazing capacity to expand to accommodate the passage of a baby. Similarly, it can contract and has enough elasticity to mold itself around a finger, a tampon, or a penis. Just inside the opening of the vagina is a ridge of muscles that tighten around the penis during intercourse. This ridge is referred to as the levator ani muscles, which are part of the pelvic floor support structures. The

Figure 3.3 Internal sex organs

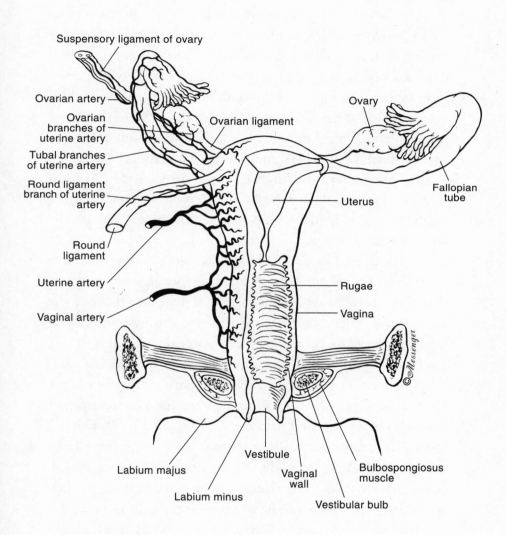

bumps or irregularities in the lining of the vagina are called
rugae. Absence of rugae in the vagina represents loss of
smooth muscle in the vaginal wall. This can occur because of

aging, menopause, or pelvic floor prolapse (see chapter 4 for more information).

The lining of the vagina is called mucosa, which is similar to the smooth skin inside your mouth. Lubrication occurs during a process called transudation: vaginal engorgement causes droplets to appear on the vaginal lining, which combine together to form a slippery fluid. Decreased vaginal lubrication, resulting in dryer vaginal walls, can occur during breast feeding, after menopause, and immediately following the menstrual period. Wetter walls occur around ovulation, during pregnancy, and during sexual arousal. The transudate allows vaginal penetration or intercourse to occur more easily and also help to keep the vagina moist, chemically balanced, and free of bacteria.

The vagina has a rich supply of blood vessels but few nerve endings except near its opening. Some women report that they are sensitive to touch only in the outer third of the vagina, but others say they are sensitive throughout, in particular to pressure on the cervix or anterior vaginal wall.

In the 1980s Alice Kahn Ladas, Beverly Whipple, and John D. Perry identified an important part of the vagina: the G-spot, or Grafenberg spot, named for the German physician who first suggested its presence in 1950. The G-spot is a mass of spongy tissue, about the size of a small bean in its unstimulated state, located in the front wall of the vagina almost directly below the urethra, or urinary opening. When stimulated, the tissue swells to the size of a dime or larger.

To find the G-spot, it is best to squat or sit and then explore the upper front wall of the vagina with your finger by applying firm, rhythmic pressure upward against the wall. The first sensation many women feel when they touch the

G-spot is a need to urinate, but the feeling usually passes as they continue to stimulate the G-spot to the point that it swells to a small lump. Continued stimulation brings some women to intense orgasms that they feel deeper inside the vagina than they do clitoral orgasms. Generally, we've found from our patients that G-spot orgasms are more difficult to achieve than clitoral orgasms. Most partners also need to be told where to find the spot. Manual stimulation by a partner is one way to reach a G-spot orgasm, often with three or four fingers, but other women say rear-entry or a woman-on-top intercourse position with a patient partner works well also. (See chapter 9 for more information.)

Cervix: The cervix is the small round structure at the upper end of the vagina that is the opening into the uterus, or the "mouth" of the womb. If you haven't had a baby, the cervix looks like a smooth, fleshy button with a small hole in the center, almost like a doughnut. The opening, or os, is about the same diameter as a very thin straw. Sperm passes through the hole and menstrual blood flows out of it, but it is far too small for a finger or a tampon. During delivery it expands to accommodate the passage of a baby up to 12 centimeters wide.

You can feel the cervix if you insert your finger up to the end of the vagina, although some days you may barely be able to touch it. On other days it may seem to have shifted position. This is in fact exactly what has happened, since the cervix changes position along with the natural changes in position and shape of the uterus from menstruation or sexual stimulation.

Glands inside the cervix produce mucus, which covers

the cervix with a coating that keeps bacteria from entering the uterus. The consistency of the cervical mucus varies, but it dissolves every month to allow for the outflow of menstrual blood.

The cervix has no nerve endings but is sensitive to pressure and movement. Some women find it painful to have a penis thrusting against the cervix, but for others rhythmic pressure on the cervix is essential to orgasm. Some women experience orgasm from this method alone. It requires deep penetration.

Uterus: The uterus is a hollow, very muscular organ about the size and shape of an inverted pear, usually about three inches long and two inches wide, located behind the bladder. Its walls are made of some of the strongest muscles in the body, which are able to contract so powerfully during labor that they push open the cervix and send the baby down the birth canal. The interior walls of the uterus are lined with endometrium, a soft, spongy tissue that builds up each month in anticipation of receiving and nourishing a fertilized egg toward pregnancy, but which is usually shed with each menstrual cycle. The walls of the uterus normally touch each other, but are pushed apart by a growing fetus. The uterus has an amazing ability to expand to accommodate a growing baby, but slowly returns to its normal size and shape after a pregnancy. Benign muscular tumors, called fibroidenomas or fibroids, sometimes grow in the wall of the uterus and may cause pain or discomfort. During orgasm, some women describe rhythmic, involuntary, and pleasurable muscular contractions of the uterus. We are currently investigating the nerves to the uterus and vagina, and what role the uterus plays in the orgasmic response.

Ovaries: The two ovaries, or female gonads, are about the size of unshelled almonds and are located on each side of the uterus, about four or five inches below your waist. They are held in place by connective tissue and have two all-important functions. One is to produce the sex hormones estrogen, progesterone, and testosterone, which plays a central role in a woman's sexual desire. The other job of the ovaries is to produce and release eggs.

The eggs in the ovaries are held inside tiny cavities called follicles. Each woman is born with about a million follicles, each containing an immature egg, but they degenerate during childhood and by the time of the first menstrual period only about 400,000 are left. Each month during a woman's reproductive years about 10 to 20 follicles begin maturing. During ovulation, usually one follicle develops enough to rupture the surface of the ovary. Since a woman's reproductive years stretch for only half her life, roughly the four decades from age 11 or 12 to slightly past 50, less than 500 eggs, or a dozen a year, are involved in ovulation and have a chance at fertilization and developing into a baby. (See chapter 6 for more information about changes in women's sexual function throughout the life cycle.) A man, by contrast, produces sperm throughout his entire life.

Fallopian Tubes: The two fallopian tubes, or oviducts—literally, "egg tubes"—are each four to five inches long and extend outward from the upper end of the uterus toward the ovaries. One description we like, from *Our Bodies, Ourselves,* likens them to ram's horns facing backward. The inside lining of the tubes is covered by cilia, which are hairlike, microscopic outgrowths. The far ends of the fallopian tubes flare out in very delicate fingerlike extensions called fimbria, which sit near the ovaries but are not attached to them. These tubes may become blocked by infection, impairing a woman's ability to conceive normally.

At the time of ovulation, which normally occurs on alternating sides each month, the egg is released from an ovary but floats freely in the small gap between the ovary and fallopian tube until the fimbria successfully sweep it into the tube. The egg then spends several days in the fallopian tube on its journey toward the uterus. Wavelike contractions of the muscles in the tube and movements of the cilia propel the egg onward. This generally occurs between days 14 and 17 of the menstrual cycle. If the egg is to meet with sperm, it usually does so in the upper portion of the fallopian tube. From there the fertilized egg continues toward the uterus, where it will implant in the endometrium and, if all goes well, develop into a fetus. Rarely, a fertilized egg in the tube will be unable to pass, causing a tubal, or ectopic, pregnancy. An unfertilized egg eventually disintegrates and will be washed out unnoticed in the menstrual flow.

Other Parts of the Sexual Anatomy

Breasts: For all of their allure in Western society, the breasts are simply modified sweat glands surrounded by fatty, fibrous tissue (although they do have a vital function, to provide nourishment to the infant). Erotic sensitivity in the breasts varies enormously. Studies are under way to better evaluate "normal" breast and nipple sensation as well as the variables involved in the loss of nipple sensation with aging, menopause, and surgery. Many women experience little feeling when their breasts are caressed, but for others the breasts are a source of great sexual pleasure. For many women the most erotic part of the breast is the nipple, which has a network of nerve endings that make it highly sensitive to touch. Around the nipple on the flat surface of the breast is the areola, which is the circle of dark skin with many nerve and muscle fibers that cause the nipple to stiffen and become erect. In some women, stimulation of the nipple and areola, whether by a partner's tongue or a finger, can lead directly to orgasm. Some women describe a pleasurable sensation when nursing. The size of the breasts has nothing to do with how a woman responds, but studies have shown that women with larger breasts have less nipple and breast sensation than women with smaller breasts. Breast reduction surgery can have both negative and positive impacts on breast and nipple sensation. Some women happily report enhanced sensation, while others describe the enhanced sensation as irritating or unpleasant.

Anus, rectum, and buttocks: The anus, rectum, and buttocks can be erotic areas in many women. The anus is particularly sensitive to touch, and stimulation of it can be a part of foreplay. Some women also find the insertion of a finger into the anus and rectum arousing during foreplay or intercourse. Some women find anal intercourse highly arousing as well, while others find it painful and unpleasant. It has dangerous risks, since, unlike the vaginal lining, the delicate lining of the rectum is easily torn and can provide an entry into the bloodstream for the virus that causes AIDS and other sexually transmitted diseases. It can also be dangerous passing germs from the rectum to the vagina if vaginal intercourse occurs immediately after anal intercourse. The penetrating partner should always wash thoroughly before making such transitions and should always use a well-lubricated condom for anal penetration because the tissue of the rectum can tear or be injured. The buttocks have relatively few nerve endings, but they often respond to strong stimulation like massage or kneading. Many societies, including ours, consider them as erotic as breasts.

Physiological Mechanism for Orgasm and Arousal

Most of what we know about the mechanics of orgasm and arousal stems from the pioneering work of Masters and Johnson, who in the 1950s and 1960s observed nearly 700 men and women engaged in intercourse or masturbation in their laboratory at Washington University Medical School in St. Louis. Until then, sexual response had been studied only in animals. Although Alfred Kinsey had interviewed thousands of men and women about their sexual practices, Masters and Johnson were the first to record the observable physical details of human sexual arousal. From these observations they developed a standard model of sexual response, which they said occurred in four phases: excitement, plateau, climax, and resolution.

In the three decades since, some critics have called the Masters and Johnson model flawed, saying that the observations were made in an artificial setting, that the participants were not reflective of the general population (the initial participants were male and female prostitutes), and that the results were too focused on the genitals and penis-to-vagina intercourse. More recent researchers, like the psychiatrist and sex therapist Helen Singer Kaplan, have expanded on the Masters and Johnson model to include the emotional aspects of sex and the connection, especially for women, between the mind and the body. In Kaplan's view, desire is the first and most important phase, which is then followed by arousal and orgasm.

Dr. Rosemary Basson, a researcher at Vancouver General Hospital and the director of the first large-scale placebo-controlled study of sildenafil in women, sees the Masters and Johnson model of sexual response as only one variant of female arousal and orgasm. The female sexual response, she says, can't always be drawn as a simple mountain with a peak that represents orgasm. Basson has shown that some sexually healthy women draw a line that looks like gentle hills to represent their sexual response, with no specific peak; other sexually healthy women draw a mountain range of multiple peaks. Like Kaplan, Basson also views desire as the first phase of the female sexual response, but she calls it a "motivational force" that drives a woman to seek out sex for reasons that are not necessarily connected to physical pleasure. A woman may feel desire to have sex to increase emotional intimacy, for example, or to show affection, or to give something of herself to her partner. Dr. Basson's work has been instrumental in forwarding our understanding of the psychological aspects of female sexuality and response.

Only recently, researchers like ourselves are expanding medically and physiologically on the Masters and Johnson model, using new technologies such as photoplethysmography and Duplex Doppler ultrasound to evaluate a woman's genital blood flow during arousal. Dr. Roy J. Levin of the University of Sheffield in England is a physiologist who has been doing research in this field for many years. He and his

Figure 3.4 Pubococcygeus muscle

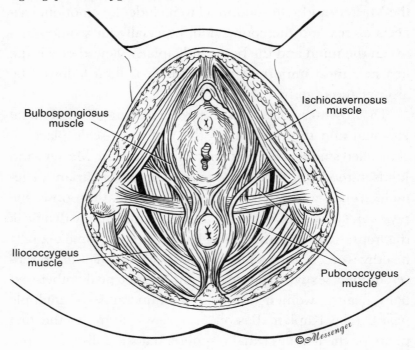

Bulbospongiosus
muscle

Ischiocavernosus
muscle

Iliococcygeus
muscle

Pubococcygeus
muscle

©Messenger

team have recorded vaginal changes during arousal and orgasm by measuring the contractions and pressures of the
genital muscles. Although the new research has confirmed
many features of the Masters and Johnson model, it has also
shown that a monolithic model of sexual response is much
too limited in its approach.

Here is what we know happens physiologically to women
during sexual arousal and orgasm: When a woman is sexually excited or stimulated, the first change to occur is an increase in blood flow to the genitals, which she may notice as
a feeling of pressure or fullness in her pelvis. At the same
time she may notice a twitching of the pubococcygeus, or
pc, muscles (see figure 3.4). Many women consciously or un-

consciously flex these muscles whenever they feel aroused. Lubrication of the vagina begins a short time later, sometimes as soon as 30 seconds after the beginning of sexual stimulation. Vaginal lubrication occurs because the increased blood flow to the vagina triggers a process called transudation, or a seeping of moisture across the vaginal lining. As lubrication increases, it sometimes flows out of the vagina, making insertion of the penis into the vagina smoother and easier.

Meanwhile, the extra blood flow causes the upper two-thirds of the vagina to balloon, the uterus and cervix to expand, and the clitoris to enlarge. The extra blood also causes the lower third of the vagina to swell, narrowing the vaginal

Figure 3.5 Blood flow to the genitals, pre-aroused

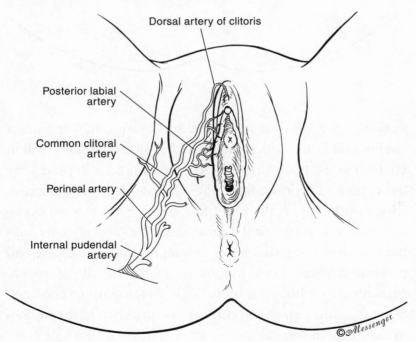

Figure 3.6 Blood flow to the genitals, aroused

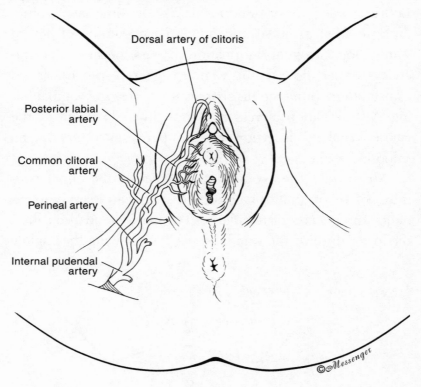

opening by a third or more and so ensuring that the outer vagina and labia, which have also become engorged, will in effect grip the penis upon insertion and hold it in place, like brake pads. The inner lips double or even triple in thickness, which pushes apart the outer lips, making the vaginal opening more accessible. At the same time, the clitoral glans pulls back against the pubic bone, retracting under its hood and protecting itself from the overintensity of direct touch. Muscles throughout the body begin to tense up or contract, heart rate and respiration come more quickly, and the nipples usually become erect.

Orgasm is reached when stimulation of the clitoris or pressure on the vaginal wall or cervix causes body tension and pelvic engorgement to build to a climax. Rhythmic and pleasurable contractions of the uterus, the outer third of the vagina, and the anal sphincter expel blood flow from the pelvic tissues back into circulation. Masters and Johnson described the first few orgasmic contractions as intense and close together, with the rest diminishing in force and duration. A mild orgasm, they said, may have only five contractions, while an intense orgasm may have as many as 15.

Figure 3.7 Nerves to the genitals

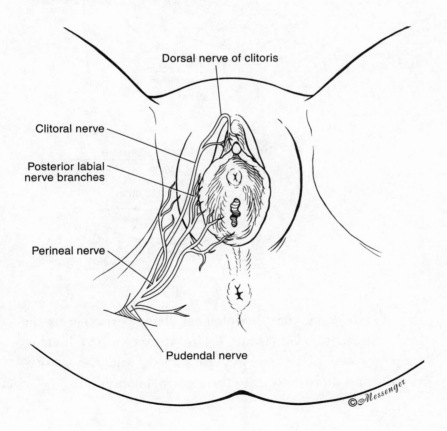

Dorsal nerve of clitoris

Clitoral nerve

Posterior labial nerve branches

Perineal nerve

Pudendal nerve

©Messenger

Figure 3.8 Pelvic organs and arteries, pre-aroused (side view)

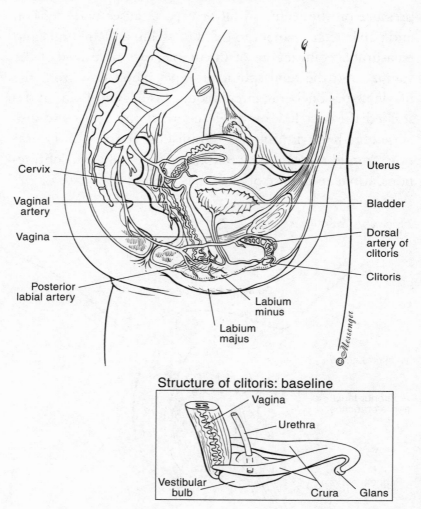

Cervix

Vaginal artery

Vagina

Posterior labial artery

Uterus

Bladder

Dorsal artery of clitoris

Clitoris

Labium minus

Labium majus

©Messenger

Structure of clitoris: baseline

Vagina

Urethra

Vestibular bulb

Crura

Glans

After orgasm, the physiological changes reverse as the body returns to a nonaroused state. It takes a half hour or more for the pelvic swelling to subside and the clitoris, vagina, and uterus return to their normal condition.

Generally, women can be multiorgasmic, which means that some can have one or more orgasms shortly after the first one—unlike men, who have what is called a refractory period immediately after climax, when the penis becomes flaccid and further stimulation is required for an erection to resume and orgasm to occur. Multiple orgasms in women also depend, of course, on continued sexual stimulation. Sometimes a woman who has a vaginal orgasm with intercourse can then have her partner stimulate her for one or more clitoral orgasms afterward. Other women have one orgasm and are satisfied. This is not to say that pleasurable sex has to include orgasm at all.

Some women experience something called female ejaculation, which occurs right before, during, or just following orgasm. Many experts report that all women can learn to ejaculate, but some do it spontaneously. Women who do ejaculate and don't understand that it is a normal variable of sexual response may feel shame and embarrassment, believing that they are urinating. Indeed, the ejaculate comes from the urethra, but when analyzed has been found not to be urine. Many believe it is fluid from the Skenes gland, an internal gland located at the same place as the G-spot. Ejaculation is thought to occur as a result of G-spot stimulation alone or in combination with clitoral stimulation. The important thing to remember is that female ejaculation is perfectly normal. Although ejaculation is certainly not necessary for a woman to achieve sexual satisfaction, it is simply one more erotic potential that she may wish to explore. (See chapter 9 for more information.)

One important subject that Masters and Johnson did not address was the difference in orgasms—a controversial topic

Figure 3.9 Pelvic organs and arteries, aroused (side view)

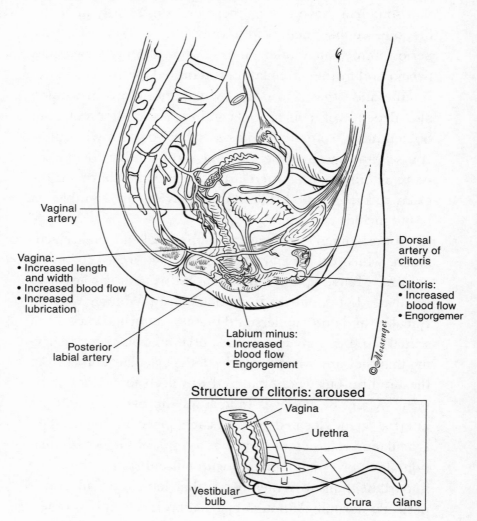

Vaginal artery

Vagina:
• Increased length and width
• Increased blood flow
• Increased lubrication

Posterior labial artery

Labium minus:
• Increased blood flow
• Engorgement

Dorsal artery of clitoris

Clitoris:
• Increased blood flow
• Engorgemer

©*Messenger*

Structure of clitoris: aroused

Vagina

Urethra

Vestibular bulb

Crura   Glans

that has divided sex researchers since Freud, who believed that the vagina was the center of the mature woman's sexual response. Freud viewed the penis as central to a woman's sexual pleasure, and pushed many "neurotic" women who did not have vaginal orgasms into psychoanalysis. Masters and Johnson, in contrast, said that all female orgasms were essentially clitoral. Even during intercourse, they said, it was the rubbing of the pelvis against the clitoral hood or traction on the pelvis that brought a woman to orgasm.

For our purposes, we quantify orgasms into two groups, clitoral and pelvic floor. Clitoral orgasms come from direct stimulation of the clitoris and surrounding tissue. The pelvic floor orgasms include G-spot orgasms and those reached by pressure on either the cervix, the anterior vaginal wall, or both. An orgasm can also be a blended orgasm, or a combination of the two. As we can't say too often, one kind of orgasm is no better than another, and orgasms do not have to be a central part of a woman's sexual satisfaction. For many couples, the intimacy, exploration, sensuality, and connection of sex can be lost when it becomes goal-oriented, focusing on orgasm as the ultimate sexual experience.

Doctors Marcia and Lisa Douglass, the authors of *Are We Having Fun Yet?*, acknowledge the importance of what they call the Cligeva, the combination of the clitoris, G-spot, urethra, and vagina. The name suggests the order in which most women enjoy their genitals to be stimulated: clitoris, G-spot, vaginal penetration, using the pc muscles to bring all the parts of the Cligeva together. They also refer to the "U-spot," the area around the urethra, as an erogenous zone.

A large percentage of women have only clitoral orgasms, through either manual or oral stimulation, and many need more stimulation of the clitoris than just the thrusting of the penis. A survey by Carol Rinkleib Ellison in her book *Women's Sexualities* found that 38 percent of 2,600 women studied have not once had an orgasm during intercourse. Many women reach orgasm before or after intercourse, or without intercourse at all. Although most women are satisfied with clitoral orgasms, we have some patients who come to us worried that clitoral stimulation is the only way they are able to reach orgasm—even if they're having those orgasms during intercourse. They think this is abnormal. Our goal is to reassure them about normalcy but also to teach them about different positions as well as the G-spot and how they may enhance their sexual response and satisfaction.

We also recommend Kegel exercises to strengthen the pelvic floor muscles. This exercise involves tightening the vagina and buttocks as if you were trying to stop urine flow or gas from being expelled. In addition to preventing and improving symptoms of incontinence, these exercises can improve orgasm response and allow for vaginal orgasms. We'll talk more about those in chapter 9.*

---

*We are beginning a study evaluating the effects of stimulation of the pudendal nerves on orgasm response. Women sit in a special chair that has been developed by Neotonus, Inc., for improving pelvic floor muscle tone. They will be receiving treatments over a six-week period. See our Web page at newshe.com for more information and the results of this study.

CHAPTER FOUR

Female Sexual Dysfunction: Definitions and Causes

Her sex drive was "in the cellar," Susan told us, and she felt "dead from the waist down." She hadn't had an orgasm in three years, ever since a doctor had performed an exploratory laparoscopy to investigate abnormal bleeding in her uterus. Afterward a gynecologist had told Susan, a 32-year-old secretary in a large East Coast city, that her lack of desire might be the result of birth control pills. But that diagnosis didn't make sense. Even though oral contraceptives can adversely affect libido, Susan had taken them for years before the laparoscopy without negative sexual side effects. We felt there were probably more factors contributing to the problem.

Mostly Susan avoided sex with her husband because it was so frustrating. When they did have sex, she described a feeling of numbness in her genitals. "I would just lay there and feel like, 'Oh, my God, this is what it must feel like to be raped,'" she said. She had been afraid to tell her husband about her response problems or the fact that she had been faking orgasms for three years—"You've got to be delicate with the male ego," she said. Like a lot of women, Susan felt very uncomfortable talking to her husband about her sexual needs and feelings. And because she wasn't communicating with him about her difficulties and why she was no longer interested in sex, he felt increasingly angry and rejected and even thought she was having an affair. She finally confided her difficulties to him when she scheduled her appointment with us. But by that time, their relationship was in crisis.

"Maybe it's in my head," she said, which is unfortunately something too many women have been told by physicians and other caregivers for too long.

Our examination confirmed that her problems were not solely rooted in emotional issues or the conflicts of her relationship. In reviewing her history, we learned that her laparoscopy had been complicated by an injury to one of the two large arteries leading to her uterus. Although the injury was repaired, we suspected the blood flow to her genital area was diminished. After a full evaluation, we found that indeed she had low genital blood flow as well as low genital sensation. This resulted in decreased lubrication and engorgement during sexual activity. She had stopped taking birth control pills several months prior to coming to see us, and her hormone levels were all normal. Quite possibly nerve damage may have occurred as well, which would explain her sensation problems. We decided to try sildenafil to help improve her blood flow. This would potentially enhance Susan's sexual arousal, her vaginal lubrication, and her genital sensation. Susan had her first orgasm in years.

"It was like, 'Oh, my God,'" she told us afterward. "Because I wasn't expecting it." After finally telling her husband the truth, they had to work together a great deal to mend the communication gap and to help both of them get over their anger. He was angry at her for hiding her sexual response problems, but overall, things began improving at home.

In time, Susan stopped taking the sildenafil because of its side effects, its expense, and her realization that her relationship with her husband also needed work. Her sexual problems were multifaceted, and not responsive to a quick fix. Although her central problem was clearly her body, not her mind, each was typically playing against the other. Sildenafil, however successful, can sometimes mask larger problems in a marriage. For this reason, Laura recommended counseling and referred Susan and her husband to a respected sex therapist in their city. The therapist encouraged more communication between the two and emphasized massage and other kinds of sensual touching during foreplay, and made the point, as we always do, that there is much more to sex and intimacy than intercourse and orgasm. Susan now tells us that the therapy has helped a great deal and has allowed her to talk more openly with her husband. Still, the physiological problem with blood flow to her pelvis continues. Now that her relationship issues are on their way toward resolution, Susan is thinking of using sildenafil again.

Susan said the main drawbacks to sildenafil were the accompanying head congestion and temporary blue tinge to her vision, which are not common to everyone. She has also been shocked that Viagra, the name under which sildenafil is marketed, is $10 a pill. (It isn't covered by her insurance because the Food and Drug Administration has not yet approved Viagra for women. Some health plans cover Viagra prescriptions for men.) More to the point, she was embarrassed to go to the pharmacy to pick it up. When the woman pharmacist told her that she owed $150, "I almost fainted," Susan said, which caused the pharmacist to ask, in a disapproving tone, "Do you still want it?" Susan quietly told her that she did.

Susan's diagnosis of sexual dysfunction encompasses a variety of disorders specific to women, such as hypoactive sexual desire disorder and sexual arousal disorder. These conditions were identified by the American Psychiatric Association two decades ago. But it wasn't until 1998 that a multidisciplinary consensus panel met in Boston and redefined these disorders, saying for the first time that medical problems can be a cause of sexual dysfunction. The goal of the panel was to create uniform standards in an exploding field, but we've also learned from our patients that it's a relief for them to have a medical basis for conditions that women were so often told were all in their heads. (Even so, we prefer the term "female sexual dissatisfaction" when we talk to our patients. It seems too much of a stigma to label someone as dysfunctional when so many women suffer from these complaints.)

In order for a woman to be considered to have a "sexual disorder," the symptoms must be persistent and pervasive and her problem must cause *her* personal distress. If it's bothering only her partner, then by definition she does not have sexual dysfunction. All the disorders can be either primary, meaning the problem has always been there, or secondary, meaning that the woman was satisfied at one point with her sexual function but no longer is.

The consensus panel was sponsored by the Sexual Function Health Council of the American Foundation for Urologic Disease.* A group of 19 experts from five countries,

---

*This is the same foundation that funded Jennifer's two-year research project on the physiology of vaginal and clitoral smooth muscle structure and function.

including Jennifer, built on the existing definitions of female sexual dysfunction to make sure that a range of different disciplines would use the same definitions and the same vocabulary. Members of the panel included gynecologists, urologists, psychiatrists, psychologists, endocrinologists, and pharmacologists. After 17 hours hours of discussion and debate, the panel unanimously approved the following four classifications of female sexual dysfunction, which are quickly becoming standard in our field. These classifications are subtyped as lifelong or acquired (new onset); generalized (happens all the time) or situational (happens only under certain conditions); and organic (due to a medical disorder) or psychogenic; or mixed. All of these disorders may occur alone or in combination requiring one or a number of treatment approaches, which we discuss at length in chapter 5. The classifications follow.

1. ***Hypoactive sexual desire disorder:*** A lack of sexual desire that causes a woman personal distress. This includes a persistent or recurring deficiency or absence of sexual fantasies or thoughts, or a lack of interest in sexual activity. As a subcategory, it includes sexual aversion disorder. Hypoactive sexual desire disorder may be the result of medical factors (such as medications), emotional factors (such as depression), or menopause (either natural or surgical). Sexual aversion disorder is the complete avoidance of sexual intercourse or relations. It is also classified as a phobic disorder that can result from physical or sexual abuse or childhood trauma.

2. ***Sexual arousal disorder:*** An inability to attain or maintain adequate genital lubrication, swelling, or other

somatic responses, such as nipple sensitivity. Disorders of arousal include a lack of vaginal lubrication; decreased clitoral and labial sensation; decreased clitoral and labial engorgement; or a lack of vaginal lengthening, dilation, and arousal. Although these conditions can be caused by psychological factors, such as depression, they can also have a medical basis, such as diminished vaginal or clitoral blood flow. Some women with physically based sexual function problems understandably develop psychological problems, which must also be addressed.

3. ***Orgasmic disorder:*** A difficulty or inability to reach orgasm after sufficient sexual stimulation and arousal. Orgasmic disorder also includes any difficulty or delay in reaching orgasm that causes the woman personal distress. The quality of the orgasm may also be diminished. Some women with orgasmic disorder describe their orgasms as "muffled," particularly if they have had strong orgasms in the past. Orgasmic disorder is most often categorized as primary, meaning that a woman has never achieved orgasm, or secondary, meaning that she can no longer achieve orgasm because of surgery, hormone deficiencies, or trauma. Primary orgasmic disorder can be caused by emotional trauma or sexual abuse, but many medical factors, such as medications or damage to the pelvic nerves during surgery, may also contribute to the problem. Clitoridectomy, or the removal of the clitoris, as practiced in some cultures in Africa, the Middle East, and Asia, would seem to be a natural cause of this category of dysfunction.

4. ***Sexual pain disorders:*** These include dyspareunia, which is recurrent or persistent genital pain associated with sexual intercourse. Dyspareunia can develop as a result of medical problems, such as vaginal infections or thinning of the vaginal lining during menopause, or following some vaginal and vulvar surgical procedures. It can also be psychologically based or reflect a relationship problem or other emotional conflict. More often than not, as with most disorders, it is a combination of physiological and psychological factors. Another sexual pain disorder is vaginismus, or involuntary muscle spasms of the lower third of the vagina, which interferes with or precludes vaginal penetration. Vaginismus usually develops as a conditioned response to painful penetration, but it can also be due to emotional or relationship problems. The panel identified a third subcategory as other sexual pain disorders, or genital pain induced by noncoital sexual stimulation. This is pain that occurs with any type of sexual stimulation other than intercourse. Although sexual stimulation triggers the pain, the primary cause of the pain can include vaginal infections, prior genital mutilation (a rite of female passage in some African countries which we discuss in chapter 6), or vestibulitis, a recurring inflammation and burning sensation around the opening of the vagina.

At our clinic we treat the full spectrum of these disorders and find that they often overlap. A woman with sexual arousal disorder, for example, may also experience orgasmic disorder or hypoactive sexual desire disorder as a result of the arousal problem. The causes are typically a combination of medical, emotional, and relationship problems that interact simultaneously—each a part of a woman's sexual pie chart, as we explained in chapter 1. Every woman is her own unique pie with the pieces divided differently, but the myriad causes of sexual dysfunction are standard, even if they are not yet widely understood.

Medical and Physiologic Problems That Can Cause Female Sexual Dysfunction

Pelvic Surgery or Trauma

Any major pelvic surgery or injury has the potential for damaging the nerves and blood vessels leading to the vagina, uterus, and clitoris. If this happens, the blood flow through the arteries may be diminished or cut off entirely, leading to a loss of sexual sensation and a reduced ability to become sexually aroused. At present, surgeons simply don't know enough about the location of the nerves and blood vessels in the female pelvis that are vital to normal sexual function to avoid severing or damaging them during surgery. Although a major plexus of nerves along the cervix, rectum, and vagina (cervical and uterovaginal plexuses) has been identified, little is known about how they connect to the clitoris and vagina. The same is not true of men: research has shown that there is a cluster of important nerves along the lateral side of the prostate. During prostate operations, surgeons take great care to preserve them, and use magnifying glasses on occasion to carefully dissect around those nerves responsible for erections. The same kind of meticulous dissection is not yet extended to women.

Hysterectomy, or the removal of a woman's uterus along with the cervix, is the second most common pelvic operation in women, after cesarean section. Approximately 600,000 are performed a year. Gynecologists report that hysterectomy should not negatively affect a woman's sexual response; in fact, they frequently suggest that her sexual response will improve. Many women do say that their sexual response improves after a hysterectomy, probably because the operation can alleviate pain caused by uterine fibroids, bleeding, and other conditions, causing women to feel healthier and thus more interested in participating in sexual activity. Women also report greater sexual freedom and pleasure because the threat of pregnancy is gone. But some women who have had hysterectomies report sexual problems afterward.

The research provides conflicting and contradictory data. Some studies report positive and some report negative sexual outcomes after hysterectomy, but no study has shown 100 percent positive or 100 percent negative results. We believe that injury to the uterovaginal and cervical plexus during hysterectomy may have an adverse effect on sexual arousal and orgasm. In addition, hysterectomy may cause sexual arousal problems by affecting lubrication and sensation. Some women describe a feeling of numbness in their vaginas during sexual stimulation. Since cervical mucus secretions contribute to lubrication, which occurs during sexual arousal as a result of vasocongestion and an increase in blood flow, removal of the cervix may cause a decrease in lubrication. Also, injury to nerves can affect blood flow and lubrication. The impact of hysterectomy on genital sensation may be due to possible damage of the uterovaginal nerves by surgery to the pelvic floor and, to a greater extent, by total hysterectomy. Hysterectomy can also result in abnormalities in the shape of the vaginal canal. Also, formation of scar tissue in the cuff (the portion of the vagina in the area where the cervix used to be), as well as a shortening of the vaginal canal, which can make intercourse painful. (See figure 5.2.)

In some women, removal of the uterus, and particularly the cervix, diminishes or eliminates the ability to have the kind of pelvic floor orgasms that come from deep vaginal penetration and cervical stimulation. Women who primarily had clitoral orgasms prior to surgery don't seem to notice the same loss. Some studies have indicated that doing what's called a supracervical hysterectomy, which leaves the cervix intact, can help maintain sexual function. However, just as many studies say the supracervical hysterectomy makes no difference. There is in fact a risk of cervical cancer in leaving the cervix in place, and no doctor would perform a supracervical hysterectomy if a woman has or has had uterine cancer. The supracervical is indicated only for women who have hysterectomies because of fibroids, benign tumors, or endometriosis.

Intuitively, leaving the cervix in may be beneficial, because we know that a large number of nerves and blood vessels are situated around it. Granted, everything above the cervix and a lot of blood vessels are still taken out.

Some doctors recommend that the ovaries also be removed in a hysterectomy, particularly in women over the age of 45 who have a family history of ovarian cancer. This removes a woman's source of estrogen and testosterone and induces menopause. Doctors will usually prescribe estrogen afterward as part of hormone replacement therapy, but not always and often without testosterone. Even if they do, there still may be an imbalance in hormone levels, affecting sexual function, which we will address later in this chapter.

Research is ongoing, but we believe that a woman's ability to enjoy sex after a pelvic operation depends in part on the extent of the surgery as well as her preoperative level of sensation and function. Clearly, a total hysterectomy has a greater chance to cause damage to blood vessels and nerves than a less invasive procedure to remove a cyst on an ovary.

Another form of pelvic surgery that may affect sexual function is a relatively new technique called uterine embolization. It is a less invasive alternative to a hysterectomy and is generally suggested for treatment of uterine fibroids, which are benign tumors that invade the walls of the uterus and can cause excessive bleeding and pain (see Endometriosis and Fibroids on pages 85–86 for more information). A doctor injects small particles of plastic, called polyvinyl alcohol or PVA, into the uterine artery, which blocks the blood supply feeding the fibroids, causing them to shrink. Like some who have undergone hysterectomy, there are some women who had prior pelvic floor orgasms who report a loss of uterine contractions and sensation after this procedure. However, the technique is being refined so that the vaginal branches of the uterine artery are spared, which might help to preserve blood flow to the vagina and pelvic floor orgasms. The UCLA Medical Center, where we have our current clinic, is one of the principal hospitals where the technique is performed. Dr. Scott Goodwin, chief of interventional radiology at UCLA, is a pioneer in the technique. The relative merits of evolving procedures, including uterine embolization or myomectomy for fibroids as well as laser or thermal-based cervical procedures, remain to be determined.

Childbirth trauma that occurs as a result of vaginal tearing from suction or forceps sometimes causes damage to the vagina as well as to the nerve and even vascular damage to the vagina and clitoris. If this occurs, problems with vaginal and clitoral sensation can develop weeks to months following the delivery. An episiotomy, a cut the doctor makes from the base of the vagina toward the anus to make it easier to deliver the baby's head, may also cause sexual problems, particularly if the incision is large or is not sewn back together appropriately. An episiotomy may take four months to fully heal.

Pelvic fractures and straddle injuries, resulting from a fall on a bicycle or a balance beam, can also cause trauma to the pubic bone and other structures in the pelvic area, including the vagina, clitoris, urethra, uterus, and bladder and their corresponding arteries and nerves.

Vasculogenic or Blood Flow Problems

Low blood flow to the pelvic organs can affect arousal, engorgement, and lubrication. We have named this disorder clitoral and vaginal vascular insufficiency syndrome, which has a variety of causes. Among the most common are:

Coronary heart disease: Coronary heart disease, or atherosclerosis, is the buildup of a fatty material called plaque along the inside walls of the arteries. The buildup narrows the arteries, and ultimately can cut off blood flow to vital organs like the heart or brain, causing a heart attack or a stroke. The same buildup can also reduce the blood flow to the arteries leading to the pelvis and genitalia, causing diminished arousal in women. In one of the studies by Jennifer and Dr. Goldstein, animals that were fed a high cholesterol diet developed atherosclerosis of their pelvic arteries and had decreased vaginal and clitoral blood flow compared to control animals.

Other studies in humans show that diminished pelvic blood flow leads to thickening and fibrosis of both the vaginal wall and the smooth muscle tissue of the clitoris. Ultimately, this can lead to symptoms of vaginal dryness and to dyspareunia. Decreased blood flow may also interfere with sexual sensation and arousal, by affecting the release of nitric oxide, and cause atrophy and degradation of nerve fibers and cells lining the vaginal canal and inner labia. This is an area of focus in our research.

High blood pressure: High blood pressure, or arterial hypertension, is an abnormal increased pressure of the blood flowing in arteries as they feed our organs and tissues. It is the most common chronic illness in the United States and can be associated with disease of the heart, kidney, and brain (stroke). In most people its cause is unknown. But excess weight, a high-fat diet, a lack of exercise, and heredity are contributing factors. High blood pressure is more common in African Americans and among younger men than younger women, but in later life women with high blood pressure outnumber men and die from it more often. More than half of all women over the age of 65 have high blood pressure.

Although high blood pressure and its treatments are known to be among the causes of male erectile dysfunction, its effect on the sex lives of women is only beginning to be understood. Just as in men, high blood pressure in women can lead to damage of the blood vessels, making them more prone to a buildup of fatty deposits and coronary heart disease. It makes sense that high blood pressure in women can be associated with decreased pelvic and genital blood flow, also contributing to decreased sexual arousal, decreased vaginal lubrication, and pain. Recently, some studies have demonstrated a correlation between a rise in blood pressure and female sexual dysfunction. The medications used to treat high blood pressure can also cause sexual dysfunction, as we discuss later in this chapter.

High cholesterol: Cholesterol is a waxy, nonsoluble substance essential to many of the body's chemical processes. It is made up of different types of fat. One type is low-density lipoprotein, or LDL, the "bad" cholesterol that allows fat to build up in the walls of the arteries. Another type is high-density lipoprotein, or HDL, the "good" cholesterol that helps remove the fatty deposits left in the arteries by carrying them to the liver, where they are broken down and secreted. Cholesterol tests measure the levels of these fats in the blood. A woman's total cholesterol level is one factor in her risk for heart disease, but doctors now think that the more important indicator is the ratio of a woman's "good" cholesterol to her total cholesterol. A woman can increase her "good" cholesterol with weight loss and regular exercise, as well as by taking certain vitamins, minerals, and maintaining a healthy diet. (See chapter 8 for more information about the effects of exercise on sexual function.)

The presence of estrogen in the blood during the childbearing years generally gives women lower cholesterol levels than men, although exactly how estrogen protects against cholesterol is unknown. After menopause, when estrogen production declines, cholesterol levels in women tend to rise, along with the risk for heart disease.

When a woman has a high level of cholesterol, excess lipoprotein deposits itself on the inside walls of her arteries, stimulating the abnormal growth of cells that scar and inflame the artery lining and leading to the formation of plaque. Large amounts of plaque can impede or cut off the blood flow to the vital organs and the pelvic region. As in the case of coronary artery disease and high blood pressure, a diminished blood flow, particularly to the vagina and clitoris, will likely reduce a woman's sexual sensation and her ability to become sexually aroused.

Smoking: Smoking causes the blood vessels to constrict, reducing the flow of blood to the heart, lower extremities, and the pelvic area. Smoking decreases the levels of estrogen and HDL, or "good" cholesterol, in the blood, both of which protect against heart disease. Toxic substances in cigarette smoke may also damage the artery walls leading to coronary heart disease.

Although few women would ever imagine that smoking might adversely affect their sex lives, the fact is that smoking, particularly heavy smoking over a lifetime, may well play a significant role in reducing blood flow to the pelvic region and can cause a woman to have a diminished sexual response. A recent study in men found that smokers with erectile dysfunction often were in the early stages of coronary disease and didn't know it. The disease affected the smallest vessels—among them, those in the penis—first.

Bicycle riding: Recent studies in men, and now in women, by Dr. Irwin Goldstein and his colleagues at Boston University and elsewhere show that prolonged riding on a standard bicycle seat may cause sexual dysfunction by crushing the bundles of nerves and arteries leading to the penis or clitoris. In one study of 282 female cyclists and 51 female runners by Michael D. LaSalle, a former fellow at Boston University's urology department who is now in private practice in New Jersey, more than 40 percent of the cyclists reported clitoral numbness while none of the runners did. (The runners served as the control group.) Interestingly, only 11 percent of the cyclists described themselves as competitive riders, and the majority wore padded bicycle shorts. Most of the cyclists used the standard narrow bicycle seat, which some experts in the field of sexual dysfunction say should be banished in favor of a wider seat—a "chair" rather than a straddle—to cause less trauma and pressure on the genitalia. The effects of extensive bicycle riding on sexual function can be permanent if the riding is prolonged over time.

Hormonal Problems

Problems related to the production of the hormones estrogen and testosterone can lead to sexual dysfunction. Some of the most frequent causes of sexual dysfunction due to hormonal factors include:

Menopause: Menopause, the cessation of a woman's menstrual periods that marks the end of her child-bearing years, occurs on average at age 51, although it can happen at any time between ages 40 and 55. Menopause is a gradual process usually lasting several years, with irregular and sometimes heavy periods that finally stop altogether. (See chapter 6 for a more detailed discussion of the effects of menopause on a woman's sexual function.) By far the most dramatic change with menopause is an enormous drop in the amount of estrogen produced by the ovaries. This loss of estrogen, the most powerful hormone in a woman's body, causes many of the common symptoms of menopause: hot flashes, vaginal dryness or irritation, incontinence, a thinning or loss of elasticity in the skin, mood swings, and depression. Many menopausal women also report a loss of libido, which is caused by a similar drop in a class of hormones called androgens. Androgens include the hormone testosterone, which is considered a "male" hormone because it is present at greater levels in men than in women. However, testosterone affects muscle strength, appetite, energy, memory, sexual desire, and response in both men and women. Hormone replacement therapy (HRT), usually estrogen and progestin, is often prescribed to counteract the effects of menopause. We are now adding testosterone to this regime. (See chapter 5 for a more detailed discussion of HRT.)

Endocrine disorders: The endocrine system is a complex network of glands that secrete the hormones that control the essential functions of the body. Disorders of the pituitary gland, an acorn-sized structure lying at the base of the brain, and the hypothalamus, a gland that is part of the brain itself, can adversely affect sexual function because they control the hormones that regulate many sexual responses. Disorders of the adrenal glands, which secrete corticosteroids that form estrogen and testosterone, can also cause sexual dysfunction. Many women with an underactive thyroid gland, a condition that causes lethargy, weight gain, aching muscles, and depression, have sexual function complaints.

Postpartum hormone deficiences: Although it is normal to experience a loss of libido in the weeks and months immediately after giving birth, usually because of exhaustion, hormone fluctuations, and vaginal soreness, a number of our patients have complained of a lack of interest in sex for years after the birth of a child. When we test their hormone levels, we often discover that they have almost no testosterone, the "male" hormone also present in women that affects sexual desire. There is limited research into why this should be the case. It may be an ovarian or adrenal failure of some sort, but a hypothesis of Laura's centers on the role of oxytocin, the hormone associated with nesting and attachment. While oxytocin is released when women breastfeed, causing a calming, pleasurable feeling, it may also be released as women immerse themselves in motherhood and the family. Oxytocin is known to suppress testosterone. Prolactin, the hormone responsible for the production of breast milk also suppresses testosterone. So as long as women are breast feeding, they will have lower testosterone levels. We also believe that some women may develop a defect in the production of testosterone, which manifests itself after childbirth. We are currently investigating this.

Diabetes: The most common endocrine disorder is diabetes, a chronic disease caused by lack of the hormone insulin or of the ability of the body to use it. Although the different types of diabetes in themselves do not necessarily affect sexual function, a diabetes-related disorder of the nervous system and blood vessels, called diabetic neuropathy, does. Neuropathy occurs in at least half of the people with diabetes. The condition, particularly common in communities of color, often causes a loss of feeling in the feet, hands, and legs. In addition to causing neuropathy, diabetes affects the small arteries to the pelvis, causing vasculogenic problems as well. Few studies have looked at the effect of diabetes on female sexual response, but those that have suggest that diabetic women do suffer from arousal as well as orgasmic difficulties.

Neurogenic Problems

Sexual function is controlled in crucial ways by the nervous system. The brain transforms sensory input—touch and sight, for example—into perceptions of pleasure or pain. In the same way, impulses sent from the brain to the body can transform sexual desire into sexual response. Many neurogenic problems can greatly disturb sexual function.

Spinal cord injury: The spinal cord links the body to the brain, and an injury—as might occur in a car, bicycle riding, diving, or industrial accident—can result in paraplegia, the paralysis of the arms or legs, or quadriplegia, the paralysis of all four limbs. There is often a significant loss of sexual function as well, depending on the severity of the injury. Women usually retain interest in sex, but may lose genital sensation and the ability to achieve orgasm. Even so, a 1996 study by Beverly Whipple, Carolyn A. Gerdes, and Barry R. Komisaruk at the State University of New Jersey showed that some women with spinal cord injury were able to experience orgasm through self-stimulation of the cervix or vagina in a laboratory setting. The women used a "passive stimulator," in essence a small rod, that was custom-made for the study. Researchers hypothesized that orgasm may have occurred via a sensory pathway that bypasses the spinal cord and carries input from the vagina or cervix directly to the brain—potentially crucial information that will help us understand the physiology of orgasm in all women.

Other women with spinal cord injury report that they can achieve orgasm with a traditional vibrator, perhaps via the vagus nerve (a nerve that fortifies the gastrointestinal tract and that can be preserved in spinal cord injury to mediate sexual response), while others say that the unaffected parts of their bodies—such as the nipples, neck, ears, or other erogenous zones—become extraordinarily sensitive, so that stimulation leads to arousal and at times orgasm. Sildenafil has also been shown to help. In a study of 19 premenopausal women with spinal cord injury at the Mount Sinai School of Medicine in New York City, a team of researchers led by Marca Sipski found significant increases in arousal among the women who took the drug and were sexually stimulated. The study, published in the June 2000 edition of the journal *Urology*, found that the maximum responses occurred when Viagra was combined with both visual and manual sexual stimulation. A placebo pill did not have the same effect.

Far more research is needed to help women with spinal cord injury or neurogenic disorders enjoy fuller sexual lives.

Other Physical Problems

Endometriosis and fibroids: Endometriosis is a condition in which the tissue that normally lines the uterus, the endometrium, grows in other areas of the body, causing pain, irregular bleeding, and often infertility. The tissue growth typically occurs in the pelvic area, on the ovaries, on the bowel, on the uterus, on the rectum, on the bladder, and in the delicate lining of the pelvis, but it can also occur in other areas of the body.

Although the cause of endometriosis is unknown, a number of theories have been proposed. Some doctors believe that endometrial cells, which are loosened during menstruation, may "back up" through the fallopian tubes into the pelvis where they implant and grow in the pelvic or abdominal cavities. Another theory suggests that a deficiency in the immune system allows menstrual tissue to implant and grow in areas other than the uterine lining. Endometriosis may also be genetic.

Once the endometrial cells implant in tissue outside of the uterus they become a problem. Each month the ovaries produce hormones that stimulate the cells of the uterine lining to multiply and swell and thicken in preparation for a fertilized egg. The endometrial cells outside of the uterus respond to this signal, but they lack the ability to separate themselves from the tissue and slough off during the next menstrual period. They sometimes bleed a little bit but they heal and are stimulated again during the next cycle. This ongoing process causes scarring and adhesions in the tubes and ovaries. These adhesions can make transfer of an egg from the ovary to the fallopian tube difficult or impossible. They can also stop passage of an egg down the fallopian tube to the uterus.

Fibroid tumors are benign tumors of muscle and connective tissue that develop within or are attached to the uterine wall. The cause of fibroid tumors of the uterus is unknown, but their growth seems to depend on regular estrogen stimulation. They show up only rarely before the age of 20 and shrink after menopause. Fibroids can be microscopic, but they can also grow to fill the uterine cavity, causing excessive bleeding and pain.

Women with either fibroids or endometriosis have a higher likelihood of suffering further complications from treatment, which can include D&C (dilation and curretage, or uterine scraping), partial or full hysterectomy, or uterine embolization (see Pelvic surgery, page 72). African-American women tend to have a higher incidence of endometriosis and fibroids than Caucasian women.

Vaginal and urinary tract infections: Infections of the vagina caused by yeast, bacteria, or parasites often result in redness, itching, burning, and an unpleasant-smelling discharge. Vulvitis, an inflammation of the vulva, is accompanied by itching, redness, and swelling. Vulvadynia, or chronic vulvar discomfort, is characterized by burning, stinging, irritation, or rawness of the vulva. Urinary tract infections, which are usually caused by bacteria that travel from the anal area to the urethra and bladder, result in intense burning upon urination. Sometimes the irritation causes blood in the urine, which is more frightening than dire, although the infections must be treated immediately. Cystitis is an inflammation of the bladder, which can be due to an infection or medication, although often the cause is unknown. The symptoms are urinary urgency, frequency, and burning. Cystitis can be treated with antibiotics if it is caused by an infection, or other medication to alleviate symptoms.

Interstitial cystitis: This is a chronic inflammatory condition of the bladder with symptoms similar to but more intense than ordinary cystitis. It is a unique form of cystitis because its causes are unknown. There is an urgent need to urinate, sometimes up to 50 times a day, with accompanying lower abdominal, vaginal, and rectal pain. The vast majority of patients are women. Urine cultures are negative and the disease does not respond to antibiotics. The disease is frequently confused with other conditions like urethral syndrome, in which women suffer from irritative bladder symptoms (urinary frequency, urgency, burning, and more) without any discernable cause, although it is sometimes associated with lesions in the bladder. To determine if a woman has interstitial cystitis, a urologist inserts a cystoscope into her urethra and looks for hemorrhages typical of the condition in her bladder. This procedure is performed while the patient is under local or general anesthesia.

We have found interstitial cystitis to be a debilitating disease that often coexists with sexual dysfunction, particularly vaginal, labial, and pelvic pain as well as arousal and orgasm problems. Research is ongoing into the causes of this problem and new medications are being developed to alleviate symptoms, but as yet there is no cure.

Pelvic floor disorders: Pelvic floor prolapse refers to relaxation and loosening of the muscles and connective tissue structures that normally hold the uterus, bladder, urethra, vagina, and rectum in their correct anatomic positions.

Prolapse can develop as a result of aging, menopause, child-birth, prolonged or traumatic labor during childbirth, as well as prior pelvic surgery (e.g., hysterectomy) and neurologic disorders. When prolapse occurs, and the supporting muscles, ligaments, and connective tissue of the pelvic floor begin to lose their supporting ability, the bladder, uterus, rectum, and even the intestines can form a type of hernia or bulge in the wall of the vagina. Each of these organs can also form a type of hernia alone or in combination with other organs. For instance, bulging or herniation of the bladder into the anterior wall of the vagina is referred to as a cystocoele, bulging of the rectum into the posterior wall of the vagina, a rectocoele, bulging of the urethra, a urethracoele, and so forth.

The most common urinary symptoms women experience as a result of pelvic floor prolapse include frequency, urgency, and incontinence. If the prolapse is severe, women will also often complain of a feeling of pressure, fullness, and pain in the vagina or rectum. Severe prolapse can be accompanied by pain in the vagina, rectum, and pelvis, as well as difficulties with bowel movements.

Aside from the urinary and bowel symptoms associated with pelvic floor prolapse, women suffering from prolapse often have sexual function complaints as well. The most typical of these sexual complaints include vaginal pain with intercourse, loss of sensation in the vagina, and difficulties with arousal and orgasm.

Jennifer has been working with Dr. Shlomo Raz, Professor of Urology at UCLA Medical Center, and one of the world's experts in female urology and pelvic floor reconstructive surgery. At present, he and Jennifer are evaluating the effects on sexual function and response of the surgeries they routinely perform to correct pelvic floor prolapse. The goal of the surgery is to restore the bladder, uterus, rectum, and vagina to their correct positions and functions. Jennifer and Dr. Raz are taking this a step further and are working toward making the operations for prolapse improve sexual function as well. They will be developing techniques to protect and preserve the nerves to the uterus and vagina that, they hope, will lead to less female sexual function problems following pelvic surgery. They are also establishing a new array of diagnostic and evaluation techniques to measure vaginal sensation before and after surgery.

Medications That Affect Sexual Function

Many drugs can adversely affect sexual response. Some of the most common are:

Antihypertensive agents: Traditional blood pressure lowering medications, like reserpine and guanethidine, often cause sexual dysfunction in men, along with dizziness and depression, and for this reason many doctors have moved away from them. Beta-blockers marketed under the names Inderal, Lopressor, Corgard, Blocadren, and Tenormin have fewer side effects, but many people who take them still complain of sexual dysfunction. In recent years calcium channel blockers, marketed as Adalat, Procardia, Calan, Isoptin, Verelan, Cardizem, Dilacor XR, and Tiazac, have become more popular, in part because they have less effect on sexual function.

Antidepressants: Tricyclic antidepressants like clomipramine, marketed as Anafranil, cause sexual dysfunction in nearly half of the patients who take it. Anafranil has actually been used for premature ejaculation in men because it delays orgasm. Other tricyclics, like Elavil, Tofranil, Sinequan, and Pamelor can cause dry mouth, dizziness, constipation, and lethargy. For these reasons, many people prefer Prozac, the first of a new generation of enormously effective antidepressants that have fewer unpleasant side effects. Prozac is a selective serotonin reuptake inhibitor, or SSRI, and works by enhancing the action of the brain chemical serotonin. But Prozac, like the newer SSRI Zoloft, causes sexual dysfunction—usually a delay in reaching orgasm, or an inability to reach orgasm—in as many as 60 percent of patients. Paxil, another SSRI, can cause a loss of libido.

Sedatives: These include medications like alprazolam, marketed as Xanax, and diazepam, or Valium. They are prescribed to relieve anxiety, but they can also cause a loss of sexual desire and arousal.

Neuroleptics: These include antipsychotic drugs, like Thorazine, Haldol, and Zyprexa, which cause sexual dysfunction as well as significant emotional blunting in some patients.

Anticonvulsants: Antiseizure drugs, including phenobarbital, marketed as Luminal, as well as Dilantin, Mysoline, and Tegretol, can cause sexual dysfunction.

Antiulcer drugs: Cimetidine, or Tagamet, was the first of a new class of highly effective ulcer drugs that are also used to treat serious heartburn. It works by blocking the secretion of stomach acid. Although side effects are not common, adverse reactions include impotence in men. We do not yet know the sexual function side effects in women.

Anticancer drugs: Tamoxifen, a drug prescribed to delay the recurrence of breast cancer that is marketed as Nolvadex, can cause vaginal bleeding, vaginal discharge, menstrual irregularities, genital itching, and depression. Patients on tamoxifen must be monitored for development of endometrial cancer.

Birth control pills: Many women taking birth control pills enjoy sex far more than before because they have been freed from their fear of pregnancy. But some women who take progestin-dominant pills complain of a loss of libido and vaginal dryness because of the hormone shifts caused by the pills.

TABLE 4.1

Drugs That Can Adversely Affect Sexual Response

All of the drugs outlined below have been shown to cause erection problems in men. They are also associated with sexual dysfunction in women, including decreased libido, decreased arousal, and orgasmic disorder.

Hypertensive Agents:

DRUG TYPE:	BRAND NAMES:	PRESCRIBED FOR:
Beta-adrenergic blocker	Inderal, Lopressor, Corgard, Blocadren, Tenormin	High blood pressure

DRUG TYPE:	BRAND NAMES:	PRESCRIBED FOR:
Calcium channel blocker	Adalat, Procardia, Calan, Isoptin, Verelan, Cardizem, Dilacor XR, Tiazac	High blood pressure

Antidepressants:

DRUG TYPE:	BRAND NAMES:	PRESCRIBED FOR:
Tricyclic antidepressant	Anafranil, Elavil, Tofranil, Sinequan Pamelor	Depression
Selective serotonin reuptake inhibitor (SRRI)	Prozac, Zoloft, Paxil	Depression

Sedatives:

DRUG TYPE:	BRAND NAMES:	PRESCRIBED FOR:
Antianxiety	Xanax, Valium	Anxiety

Neuroleptics:

DRUG TYPE:	BRAND NAMES:	PRESCRIBED FOR:
Antipsychotic	Thorazine, Haldol, Zyprexa	Psychotic disorders, manic phase of manic depression, severe nausea or vomiting, preoperative sedation

Anticonvulsants:

DRUG TYPE:	BRAND NAMES:	PRESCRIBED FOR:
Anticonvulsant, hypnotic	Luminal, Dilantin, Mysoline, Tegretol	Seizures

Antiulcer drugs:

DRUG TYPE:	BRAND NAMES:	PRESCRIBED FOR:
H2 receptor antagonist	Tagamet	Ulcers

Birth control pills:

DRUG TYPE:	BRAND NAMES:	PRESCRIBED FOR:
Progestin-dominant oral contraceptive	Ortho 7/7/7, Cyclen, Tricyclen	Birth control

---

Psychological Causes of Female Sexual Dysfunction

Depression and dysthymia: Depression is a serious problem that affects twice as many women as men, usually between the ages of 18 and 44. It can be caused by a chemical imbalance in the brain, severe stress, grief, family history, emotional conflict, or any combination of these factors. It often causes a loss of interest in sex. Dysthymia is a more common, subtle, and lower-grade form of depression that is not easily diagnosed, often because a woman is functioning adequately and doesn't know she has it. A woman with dysthymia may feel sad, isolated, overwhelmed, and unappreciated. She has a tendency to feel so unattractive and unloved that she doesn't want to let anyone else in and often withdraws from sex.

Stress: Many women today experience far more stress than men, particularly if they're full-time working mothers with small children. Many of today's supermoms are still expected to take on the majority of child-care responsibilities, even when working full-time. It is crucial for women and their partners to understand the importance of support and the sharing of domestic duties. Perhaps because of the stress in women's lives, some recent studies show that the rate of heart attack in women is actually catching up to that of men and may even surpass it. Stress causes a woman to have far more interest in sleep than in sex and can inhibit her ability to become aroused and reach orgasm. For a woman to feel sexual, she needs some time to nurture and pamper herself, but even chronically exhausted women are much less likely than men to put their own needs first.

Sexual or emotional abuse: Women who have been sexually or emotionally abused in childhood or adolescence often face a range of sexual difficulties. For some women, it is terror whenever they are in a sexual situation. For others it is an inability to stay "present" or connected to their partners while making love. Other women survivors report that they are able to respond sexually, but that they get to a point, usually right before orgasm, in which they say they "shut off" and hit a wall they can't seem to move through. Feelings of guilt, shame, anger, fear, anxiety, and isolation are all very common for these women.

Conversely, some women with a history of sexual abuse may become extremely promiscuous, engaging in a level of sexual activity that often impedes their ability to function socially. These women pursue multiple sexual encounters, trying to replace a lost love object or an unexplainable void inside. (See Sexual addiction on page 95 for more information.)

Reclaiming sexuality for a woman who has suffered sexual abuse is a slow process that takes an enormous amount of work. With support from a good therapist and partner, a woman with an abuse history can reach a point of resolution and reclaim her sexuality. Depression is a common form of response to the abuse, as is the use of alcohol and drugs. (See chapter 5 on treatment for sexual dysfunction as well as chapter 6 on sexuality through a woman's life cycle.)

Drug and alcohol use: Drug or alcohol abusers tend to have complicated emotional and sexual pasts. The substance abuse may allow for the numbing of the real pain, but that pain—as well as fear, anxiety, or shame—often carries into the sexual relationship. Many women who leave rehabilitation centers not only have to learn how to live sober but also how to relate sexually to others while sober. This can be quite a challenge. For many, sex can become a replacement for drugs or alcohol. For others, the emotional pain that was buried or "numbed" with the use of drugs or alcohol surfaces with sobriety and has a tremendously negative impact on sexual response. Therapy is a large part of healing. Trust and intimacy with a partner often need to be rebuilt as well.

Sexual addiction: Sexual addiction is a compulsive, driving need for sexual contact that can destroy family life, work life, and a person's ability to function. It is similar to addictions to alcohol and gambling, and is frequently treated with 12-step programs modeled after Alcoholics Anonymous. In fact it was former members of AA, who felt they also suffered from sexual addiction, who in the 1970s first established support groups for sex addicts. Mental health professionals did not recognize the condition until the 1980s, and even now there is controversy about its existence. But whether or not it should be treated as a formal disorder, there are clearly women and men who become obsessed with sex and exhibit the classic symptoms of addiction. Among the symptoms are a preoccupation with sex that interferes with normal sexual relations with a loved one and a repeated need for a "high" followed by feelings of guilt, anxiety, or depression. Women sexual addicts often seek out risky sex with strangers and have feelings of loneliness and worthlessness.

Body image and self-esteem problems: Fashion magazines promote such unrealistic images of beauty that many women feel they can't live up to them. These are the same women who turn out the lights during sex, and sometimes even while undressing. Hiding in this way from their partners affects the level of intimacy in a relationship. When a woman feels physically unattractive, she can't relax, be herself, and connect to another person. We've also found that women internalize negative cultural images about their own genitalia and worry far too much about vaginal appearance and odor. Consider some of the slang words for the penis— "love snake," "seven inches of heaven," "power rod"— compared to all the negative jokes about the female genitalia. In fact, books like *Femalia* edited by Joani Blank and *Sex for One* by Betty Dodson focus on this issue and try to counteract women's negative "genital esteem" by depicting the beauty and variation of female genitalia in photos and drawings.

Similarly, self-esteem plays an important role in a woman's sexual function. If a woman doesn't feel good about herself, or doesn't feel in control or powerful, it's extremely hard for her to let go and sexually respond to a partner. Feelings of powerlessness or worthlessness are not conducive to good sex. Having an orgasm in front of someone is one of the most vulnerable acts there is, but it's very hard to get to that vulnerable spot with a partner if you don't feel secure with yourself. It's also difficult to advocate for your sexual needs or tell your partner what you want, if you

don't feel good about yourself and deserving of sexual satisfaction.

Relationship problems: No drug will ever fix the sexual response of a woman who is in conflict with her partner.
No drug will ever fix a woman whose partner doesn't know
how to satisfy her, or a woman whose partner has a sexual
problem that affects her own stimulation, such as erectile
dysfunction and early ejaculation. A conflicted relationship
with a partner usually means there is a conflicted or nonexistent sex life. Communication problems, anger, a lack of trust,
a lack of connection, and a lack of intimacy can all adversely
affect a woman's sexual response and interest. (For more on
the sexual partner, see chapter 7.)

We've also found that couples in long-term relationships
and marriages sometimes have unrealistic expectations. In
most relationships, there is an initial infatuation stage, when
a couple can think of nothing else but each other and sex
is thrilling. But it is impossible to sustain those levels of
excitement—one simple reason is that you'd never get anything else done. When the relationship becomes more established and stable, sometimes after only a few months, most
couples in long-term relationships pass into the attachment
phase, which is a deeper level of commitment that moves the
relationship into a calmer, softer state, incorporated into the
rest of your life and no longer consuming it.

The most successful relationships maintain this attachment phase, which our society recognizes as love. Over time
the attachment may deepen, change shape, or shift depending on life events such as the birth of children. But it is built
on communication and intimacy. Unfortunately, a lot of

people confuse infatuation with love and think that once they get to the attachment phase they've fallen out of love. We see some women who are almost addicted to the infatuation stage, where sex is at the center. But in the attachment phase, sex becomes just one part of the relationship and that disappoints a lot of people. They feel they've lost the spark and the excitement. We've even had two-career couples with two children under three come in and tell us that they were worried because they were having sex only once a week. They feared there was something wrong with their relationship and that maybe the love had gone. We were happy to help them and stressed the importance of building in romantic time together. But given the circumstances, we told them it was wonderful that they still found time for sex at all.

CHAPTER FIVE

Treatment: The Combined Role of Medicine and Therapy

Medicine

The most important message of this chapter is that there is no single cure-all or magic bullet for female sexual dysfunction. Every woman, every problem, and every response is different. The options for treatment, which we explain here in detail, vary as much as the symptoms. The women who respond best to sildenafil and other blood-flow enhancing medications are women who at some point were satisfied with their sex lives, but now for whatever medical or physiologic reason—a hysterectomy, for example—are no longer able to respond as they once could. In contrast, women whose sexual response problems are related to relationship or partner issues or are rooted in unresolved histories of sexual abuse or other emotional problems are generally not candidates for medication as a first-line therapy. They are better served by counseling and therapy. Medications may play a role in the treatment but they will not resolve the problem unless the emotional issues are addressed. Menopausal women, who until recently only had the option of conventional hormone replacement therapy (estrogen and progesterone) or commercial lubricants (such as K-Y Jelly), can be greatly helped by the addition of testosterone to their hormonal regimen, as well as sildenafil (and other drugs now in trials) and devices. Many women will require more than one treatment, a combination of Viagra and testosterone cream, for example.

In our view, the complete medicalization of sexuality is not the answer. Diagnosis and treatment should ideally combine the mind *and* body in order to attend to all the components of a woman's sexual life.

It is important to remember that this is just the beginning of a new era, when improving sexual function has become a focus of pharmaceutical companies and the health care industry. "Better loving by chemistry" is the industry motto, even though chemistry is only part of the picture. Many of these drugs didn't exist five years ago, and the field continues to expand faster than anyone can track. But here is the best up-to-date, comprehensive explanation of the treatments that are currently or soon to be available for women.

Viagra (sildenafil): The little blue pill that started a national dialogue about erectile dysfunction, and the first oral impotence drug for men. Approved for men by the Food and Drug Administration in March 1998, Viagra's sales reached $1 billion in its first year. Now 200,000 prescriptions are filled each week. At this writing, more than 17 million Americans have tried Viagra—the vast majority of them men, although an increasing number are, and will be, women. Viagra has been enormously popular overseas as well. Although Pfizer, the maker of Viagra, does not release Viagra statistics by country, drug company analysts estimate that a quarter of the drug's sales have been outside the United States.

Amazingly, sildenafil was discovered by accident. In the early 1990s, Pfizer began testing it as a treatment in men for angina, the chest pains caused by a reduced supply of oxygenated blood to the heart. It didn't work, but Ian Osterloh, the doctor directing sildenafil's development, did notice that some test subjects were reporting an interesting side effect: erections. He didn't know what to make of the finding until he saw a 1992 paper in the journal *Science* describing how a chemical called nitric oxide, released from nerve endings in the penis, was crucial for erections. Since Dr. Osterloh already knew how sildenafil worked, an idea began to form in his head. The rest, of course, is sexual history.

Specifically, sildenafil in men blocks an enzyme that normally prevents erections from happening. When a normally functioning man is sexually aroused, nitric oxide is released within the penis from nerves, blood vessels, and penile erectile tissue. Following the release of nitric oxide, a cascade of reactions occur that are initiated by a substance called cyclic guanosine monophosphate, or cGMP. This in turn causes the blood vessels of the penis and the penile erectile tissue to relax and dilate, allowing blood to rush in and an erection, or tumescence, to occur. (See figure 5.1.)

Loss of an erection, or detumescence, is caused in part by the enzyme phosphodiesterase Type 5, or PDE5, which destroys cGMP. As long as a man is sexually stimulated, he makes enough cGMP to counter the suppressive effects of PDE5 and maintain his erection. But when ejaculation occurs or sexual stimulation ends, the production of cGMP drops and PDE5 takes over. The erection subsides. In a man

Figure 5.1   Male and female erectile tissue

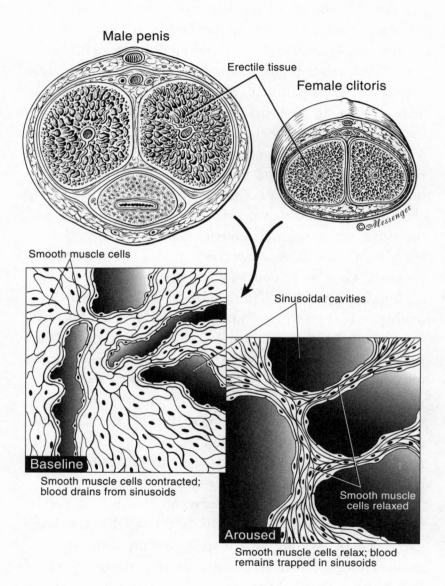

Male penis

Erectile tissue

Female clitoris

©Messenger

Smooth muscle cells

Sinusoidal cavities

Baseline

Smooth muscle cells contracted;
blood drains from sinusoids

Smooth muscle
cells relaxed

Aroused

Smooth muscle cells relax; blood
remains trapped in sinusoids

with erectile dysfunction, sildenafil works by blocking PDE5 and boosting the effects of cGMP.

Sildenafil appears to work the same way in women, leading to increased blood flow to the vagina, clitoris, and labia, causing engorgement of these tissues, enhanced sensation, and increased vaginal lubrication. However, sildenafil, will not be approved for women until the completion of clinical trials, which are now ongoing in the United States The first sildenafil trials were done only in men.

At this writing, we're helping to direct a nationwide study of sildenafil among urologists, gynecologists, psychologists, and sex therapists. This could help lead to FDA approval. The research, sponsored by Pfizer, is important because it is what's called a double-blind placebo-controlled study of a large number of women, with an extensive screening out of patients with psychological and relationship problems or with low hormone levels. Some women will be given sildenafil, others a placebo pill, and neither the researchers nor the women will know who got what—a crucial research technique for determining the actual effects of a drug that might also be working in some women because of a psychological placebo effect. We have worked a great deal in helping to determine the best candidates for the trial and in training sex therapists on how to select the best candidates for drug therapies. We've learned from our own work that women with an unresolved history of childhood sexual abuse or significant emotional or relationship issues are generally not good subjects for drug therapies as the primary intervention.

It is recommended that sildenafil be taken on an empty stomach, about an hour before intercourse, without alcohol. Planning is important; it's not the pill to take on the spur of the moment after a big anniversary dinner with lots of wine.

Also, since sildenafil works physiologically on the blood flow, and not via the brain to enhance libido, a woman (or man) must have the desire to engage in sexual relations and be sexually stimulated enough for it to have an effect. In other words, foreplay is necessary. Taking a pill and then waiting for sexual arousal to occur on its own will not work.

Headaches are the most common side effects of sildenafil, along with facial flushing, nasal congestion, and indigestion. A small number of patients also report a bluish tinge to their vision that lasts for up to a few hours after taking the pill. In addition, the Food and Drug Administration has issued warnings about reports of heart attacks, sudden cardiac deaths, and hypertension among male sildenafil users, and says that doctors should prescribe sildenafil with caution to men who have had a heart attack, stroke, or life-threatening arrhythmia in the previous six months. That said, a new study by researchers at the University of Pennsylvania published in the *New England Journal of Medicine* suggests that sildenafil causes only minor effects on blood flow in the heart. According to the study, sildenafil seems to pose no identifiable risk of heart attack apart from that caused by the exertion of sexual intercourse that sildenafil makes possible. However, people taking medicines containing nitrates, in particular the heart drug nitroglycerin, should *never* take sildenafil because the combination can cause a fatal drop in blood pressure. The FDA also cautions against giving sildenafil to men who have significantly low blood pressure, blood pressure greater than 170/110, a history of cardiac failure, unstable angina, or the eye disease retinitis pigmentosa. Although the FDA directed its warnings only at men, women should follow these precautions as well. Sildenafil should also be avoided by women who are or may want to become pregnant.

In the right patient, sildenafil can have beneficial effects, particularly in women who in the past were satisfied with their sexual response but who are now, perhaps because of menopause or a hysterectomy, experiencing problems. Lucy, for example, a 43-year-old mother of four from Mississippi, came to see us because her orgasms had changed dramatically since the removal of her uterus and ovaries 13 years earlier. "I could still have an orgasm, but it was just very weak," she said. "It was 'Why bother?'" Three doctors had told her that her weakened response had nothing to do with the hysterectomy and that her problems were probably psychological. "They told me that I should go home and work it out," Lucy told Laura. Lucy's husband, too, thought it was psychological. "He was always real quick to believe it was in my head," Lucy said. "He just felt that I didn't want sex any more. I really felt like an 'it.' It just kind of takes your identity away."

Lucy started to become depressed and eventually had to be hospitalized for what she described as a nervous breakdown. "I was just a complete basket case," she said. She recovered, but her sexual response and self-esteem did not. Like so many women suffering from sexual dysfunction, Lucy told us how she would walk down the street, be whistled at by construction workers, and feel painfully aware of how the world saw her as a sexual object. It was devastating to seem like a sexual person on the outside but to feel like a nonsexual, nonfunctioning person on the inside. At the same time, her husband was growing increasingly frustrated and feeling shut out physically and emotionally by his wife. As his feelings of rejection escalated, he withdrew from the relationship and became bitter and angry. He eventually began having an affair with a mutual friend of theirs. When Lucy discovered that her husband was having an affair with her close friend, Lucy sank into another depression that required hospitalization.

When we examined Lucy, we discovered that she had greatly diminished blood flow to her genital area. Her genital sensation was also low and her vaginal lubrication only marginal. We suspected that branches of the vaginal arteries and nerves might have been harmed during her surgery, although it was impossible to say for sure. What we can say for certain is that when we gave Lucy sildenafil during the second phase of the evaluation, she was able to have a powerful orgasm using the vibrator in our office, and in less than three minutes—the first like it in 13 years.

Laura also saw Lucy and her husband in a counseling session. The couple was still sorting out the damage from the affair and were clearly having trouble communicating. Lucy's husband felt an enormous amount of remorse; Lucy was still very angry. Restoring Lucy's sexual function seemed unlikely to repair all of the damage done to the relationship. They were going to require ongoing sex therapy and counseling, so Laura referred them to the American Association for Sex Educators, Counselors, and Therapists (AASECT), an organization that would put them in touch with a sex therapist in their area.

Since her visit, Lucy has taken Viagra regularly prior to sexual activity, which she says has restored her orgasms and improved her relationship with her husband. "It helped a lot," she said. "Because deep down, I think he felt it was a rejection of him." Most of all, Lucy seemed to feel a sense of relief that her problems were taken seriously. "There's something about being validated," she said, "after all those years of being told it's in your head."

In Lucy's case, sildenafil most likely improved her sexual response by enhancing her genital arousal and sensation. Sildenafil may increase nerve stimulation via release of nitric oxide, as it does in men. The mechanisms by which sildenafil enhances the female sexual arousal response are currently being investigated in our lab. Meanwhile, Lucy and her husband will probably continue with couples therapy in order to repair the damage done to their relationship.

Hormone replacement therapy: This is the only drug treatment currently approved by the FDA for women with complaints of sexual problems associated with the drop in hormone levels brought on by menopause. Conventional HRT, which replaces the vital hormones that a woman's ovaries no longer produce as she reaches her fifties, is highly effective in treating the symptoms of menopause, like hot flashes and vaginal dryness.

In its conventional form, HRT consists of estrogen combined with progestin, a synthetic version of the female hormone progesterone. Taking estrogen alone can cause endometrial hyperplasia, an uncontrolled growth of the uterine lining that leads to heavy bleeding. Progestin controls that growth and also protects against endometrial cancer. A woman who has had her uterus removed can take estrogen alone.

Replacement hormones alleviate symptoms of depression, improve energy levels, and provide protection against osteoporosis, or weakening of the bones, which is common in older women and responsible for hip and other bone fractures. For years, replacement hormones were believed to protect against heart disease as well, but in March 2000 researchers for an ongoing federal study of 25,000 women warned that replacement hormones may in fact put women at a slightly higher risk of heart attacks and strokes.

In addition, women who have had breast cancer should not take HRT because some breast cancers are stimulated by estrogen. Many studies show a slight increase in breast cancer among women taking replacement hormones, particularly if the hormones are taken for more than a decade. Two recent studies, one by the National Cancer Institute and the other by the University of Southern California, found even higher risks of breast cancer when a woman's hormone replacement therapy included progestin, suggesting that it was a more important factor in cancer risk than estrogen. But overall, women who take hormone replacements tend to live longer than those who do not. With so much confusing evidence, women should carefully weigh their own health and family histories when they consider HRT.

Estrogen pills, widely marketed as Premarin, the best-selling drug in the United States, are usually taken one a day for the first 25 days in a calendar month. If you tend to forget to take pills, an estrogen skin patch might be a better option. It's usually about two to three inches wide, attaches to the abdomen or buttocks, and releases a steady stream of estrogen into the body. You can shower and swim while wearing the patch, but it needs to be changed every three to five days.

Progestin is available only in pill form. It is usually taken with estrogen pills the first 10 to 14 days of the month. Progesterone prevents the endometrial lining from thickening, which reduces the risk for bleeding and endometrial tumors.

Estrogen is also available in a silicone ring called an estradiol vaginal ring, or Estring (from Pharmacia & Upjohn), which is inserted into the vagina, much like a diaphragm, for 90 days at a time. In this way estrogen is only minimally absorbed by the body. Some gynecologists will allow some women with a history of breast cancer to use Estring, depending on their histories and the types and stages of their tumors. Nonetheless, any woman with a history of breast cancer or at risk of breast cancer should check with her oncologist first. Vaginally delivered estrogen is now available in a small, film-coated tablet called Vagifem (from Pharmacia & Upjohn) that a woman inserts into her vagina once daily for two weeks, then twice a week thereafter. The tablet dissolves spontaneously and some women feel it is easier to use and less messy than the estrogen creams. These delivery systems are designed to improve local vaginal symptoms of dryness and irritation.

Some women are afraid to take hormones, based on the fact that they are not "natural" or have such side effects as breast tenderness, water retention, irregular bleeding, and monthly periods. As we emphasize throughout this book, we will consider any conventional alternative therapy that has been well studied in women, is safe, and eases symptoms of sexual dysfunction. Decreased estrogen levels are not only associated with hot flashes, osteoporosis, and urogenital symptoms, but can also cause anxiety, depression, and memory loss. For these reasons we are supporters of using HRT under the appropriate conditions. We also believe that a woman should be informed of her options and the decision to begin HRT should be made jointly with her doctor.

Menopausal women might also want to consider one of the new "designer estrogens" now on the market, raloxifene. More accurately known as a selective estrogen-receptor modulator, or SERM, raloxifene is a close cousin of tamoxifen,

a drug used to prevent breast cancer. Like tamoxifen, raloxifene is a synthetic estrogen that has also been shown to prevent breast cancer. (In 1997 a study by Eli Lilly, the maker of
the drug, found that raloxifene reduced the risk of breast
cancer by up to 70 percent in 7,700 women.) But it is marketed, under the brand name Evista, chiefly to counter postmenopausal bone loss.

Menopausal women with a history of breast cancer who
can't take estrogen can take raloxifene, although it is not a
perfect substitute. It does help to prevent osteoporosis, but it
builds up bone density at only half the rate of estrogen. It
doesn't have a beneficial effect on cholesterol levels, doesn't
help vaginal atrophy, and has no effect on hot flashes. In fact,
it may even cause them. But since it doesn't cause breast cancer and may well prevent it, there is a great deal of excitement about raloxifene. In the last few years, doctors have
begun prescribing it to menopausal women with a history of
breast cancer or to those worried about breast cancer.
Doctors also prescribe it to women who are having a relatively easy menopause but who want some protection for
their bones.

Finally, menopausal women can build up their estrogen
supply naturally by eating soy-based foods such as tofu, soy-
beans, soy milk, soy nuts, or two to three tablespoons a day of
flaxseed. A good book to consult for recipes and amounts is
Estrogen: The Natural Way by Nina Shandler. (See the
Resources section in chapter 9.) However, women need to be
warned that eating large amounts of estrogen in food without progestin as a balance may cause heavier menstrual
bleeding and endometrial cancer.

A last note on hormone replacement therapy: although
we often prescribe estrogen to our patients in combination

with other drug therapies that enhance genital blood flow, estrogen is not always completely effective in treating problems of sexual desire, arousal, and orgasm. In fact, estrogen increases a protein in the blood called steroid hormone binding globulin (SHBG), which actually binds to testosterone, causing it to become unavailable to the cells. Thus, estrogen replacement therapy alone, without testosterone, can actually lower testosterone levels in the blood. For this reason, we have found that many women receiving estrogen alone will experience a loss of libido and will need testosterone.

Testosterone: Testosterone is the hormone that affects sexual desire. It is widely considered the "male" hormone because it is responsible for masculine characteristics like facial hair and a deep voice, but it is also present in much smaller amounts in women. Like estrogen, testosterone is produced by the ovaries and adrenal glands and declines gradually throughout a woman's life. Reduced testosterone levels can create widely varying symptoms. Some women never notice the difference, while others are devastated by a sudden or gradual decline in libido.

Ironically, the estrogen in traditional hormone replacement therapy can cause a woman's testosterone level to drop even further. That's because, as we mentioned above, estrogen increases a substance in your blood called steroid hormone binding globulin, or SHBG, which binds to testosterone, making it unavailable to the body. Testosterone levels also decline by about a third in premenopausal women who have had both ovaries removed.

A number of studies have shown that testosterone does improve sexual desire and response, particularly in women who have had their ovaries removed. A study published in the *New England Journal of Medicine* in September 2000 found that the use of an experimental testosterone skin patch developed by Watson Pharmaceuticals can improve sexual response and psychological well-being in surgically menopausal women. However, testosterone is still controversial, and some health care professionals are reluctant to prescribe it. This is largely because early studies showed that given in high doses, testosterone has masculinizing side effects like increased hair growth and a deepening of the voice. It can also cause weight gain and acne. More serious side effects with high doses include an increase in cholesterol levels and the risk of liver and heart disease. Unfortunately, many doctors still think that in any dose testosterone will cause women to grow beards or become aggressive. Others are simply uninformed about the role it plays in a woman's sexuality.

To us, testosterone is so central to a woman's sexual function that no lover and no amount of sexual stimulation can make up for its absence. We have had significant success in treating our patients with testosterone and think it has a definite benefit for women with low desire and documented low testosterone levels. We have also found that testosterone and estrogen, alone or in combination, are both good treatments for pain related to atrophy or thinning of the vagina or labia. They also relieve symptoms associated with vulvitis and vulvadynia.

After the medical history, a blood test is the first step in determining whether a woman needs testosterone. We check three things: the levels of SHBG in the blood, the amount of unbound or "free" testosterone in the body, and the amount of total testosterone and dihydroepiandosterone (DHEA) levels. (DHEA is described below.) The two most important indicators are free testosterone and the ratio of free testosterone to total testosterone, since together those tell us how much testosterone is actually available to a woman. The normal range for total testosterone is usually 14 to 76 nanograms per deciliter, although Dr. Susan Rako, the author of *The Hormone of Desire,* one of the most popular books available on the importance of testosterone for women, sets normal at 20 to 50 nanograms per deciliter. We agree with her, and think that anything below 20 nanograms per deciliter is too low, indicating that testosterone therapy should be considered. One problem that women need to be aware of: blood tests are inaccurate in women who are already taking methyltestosterone, a synthetic derivative (and anabolic steroid) and so far the only form of testosterone marketed by the drug companies. Some labs have ways of detecting methyltestosterone levels in the blood, but the techniques are expensive. Also, different labs have different normal values and different ways of measuring the levels. These things need to be taken into account when evaluating a patient's testosterone levels or beginning testosterone replacement.

For postmenopausal women, methyltestosterone is available in pill form in Estratest or Estratest H.S., for "half strength." But both are fixed combinations of estrogen and methyltestosterone. Estratest H.S. contains 1.25 milligrams of methyltestosterone and .625 milligrams of estrogen, whereas full strength Estratest contains 2.5 milligrams of methyltestosterone and 1.25 milligrams of estrogen. On occasion, women will require less estrogen and more testosterone, or vice versa, making the fixed combination difficult to use. Under these circumstances, we have our compounding pharmacist Dr. Ray Burns of the Urgent Care Pharmacy in Boston formulate testosterone for us. We think an ideal dose for most women is between .25 and 2 milligrams per day. This lower dose provides benefits of increased libido and response, but less risk for negative side effects. (In higher doses it can cause high cholesterol, liver problems, acne, weight gain, and excessive hair growth in the pubic area and chest.)

Estratest is in fact a drug that is FDA approved for treatment of hot flashes. Although it is not FDA approved for treatment of loss of libido, studies are under way to assess the effects on libido under conditions of estrogen deprivation and replacement.

Physicians can get testosterone capsules for their female patients from what are called "compounding pharmacies," generally independent drugstores, not part of the big chains, that supply individualized doses of testosterone. A compounding pharmacist, always licensed, takes raw material from pharmaceutical suppliers and repackages or "compounds" it to fill prescription orders written by doctors. This was the system of the old corner drugstore before the large pharmaceutical companies began manufacturing and packaging their own drugs.

Testosterone is available from compounding pharmacies in the form of pure testosterone, testosterone propionate, testosterone ethanotate, or as the synthetic methyltestosterone. Compounding pharmacists can make testosterone doses in the form of sublingual lozenges or sprays, which unlike capsules will bypass the liver and thus eliminate the potential for liver damage. Testosterone is also available in patches or creams. Subcutaneous implants have been used in Australia and the United Kingdom, but are not available in the United States.

Susan Rako reports that there are about 2,500 compounding pharmacies out of the 65,000 in the United States. If your doctor doesn't know of one where you live, check our Resources section in chapter 9. Most compounding pharmacies will ship anywhere in the United States.

One of our patients who was greatly helped by testosterone is Margot, a 38-year-old mother of two and a Boston area nurse. She came to our clinic complaining of a total loss of sexual desire, saying that she no longer thought about sex, never experienced sexual fantasies, and sometimes felt disgust when she was touched. In addition, she said that she had always had some trouble reaching orgasm, but that the problem had steadily worsened, first after the birth of her children, then during a depression two years earlier, which she described as a "chemical thing" without apparent cause.

When in the mood, she told Laura, she generally could reach orgasm alone with a vibrator, but not with her husband— either through sexual intercourse or manual or oral stimulation. Sex was a cause of enormous frustration in her marriage—"It was pushing us apart," she said—and she and her husband were in counseling.

Our examination showed that Margot did not have any medical problems and her physiologic measurements were all normal. But when we evaluated her hormones, we found that she had very low levels of total and free testosterone. We prescribed methyltestosterone, eventually settling on a dose of 1 milligram daily.

It worked. Although reaching orgasm was still a challenge, it was easier. More important, Margot was interested in sex for the first time in years. "I can fantasize again, I dream about things, I think about it," she said. "The desire is there." Her relationship with her husband improved. Her newfound desires also made her feel less isolated and more like the other women around her. "Now I feel like I think like most of my friends," she said.

Testosterone is also available over the counter in the form of DHEA, or dehydroepiandosterone, an androgenic steroid. DHEA has been available as an energy booster in the vitamin section of pharmacies and health food stores for years. But it's only in the last year that some doctors have begun to prescribe it for low libido in women. The standard dose is 50–150 milligrams per day, taken each morning. DHEA is being tested in women at present, and in nonplacebo-controlled studies, results seem promising. However, larger scale placebo-controlled studies are needed to fully assess the effectiveness of this medication. Some women find it effective, but it often takes several months to see an effect. At this point DHEA is controversial and we rarely prescribe it as a first-line therapy. The problem is that it's not regulated by the FDA, so one can't be certain that the amount in each pill is consistent. We also don't yet know exactly how it works in the body. We strongly urge any woman considering DHEA to check with her doctor first.

Finally, an important warning: pregnant women and women trying to conceive should never take testosterone, because it can cause the fetus to develop problems with the reproductive and genital organs.

Estrogen and testosterone cream: We find these effective in many patients, particularly those who need more help with lubrication and sensation. For women who are taking estrogen orally but who are still having significant vaginal dryness and discomfort, we often consider adding the cream. It's important to point out, however, that estrogen, in the form of estradiol, does get absorbed into the body. The cream, available as Estrace or Premarin, is applied with an applicator directly inside the vagina once a day. Because the amount of estrogen absorbed by the body can be significant, women with a history of blood clots or breast or endometrial cancer should not use the cream. Women who only have symptoms of vaginal irritation and/or dryness should consider Estring or Vagifem, which deliver a continuous low dose of estrogen locally to the vaginal tissue.

Testosterone cream is applied in a small amount to the clitoris and inner labia to help improve sensation. It also helps build up thin, atrophic genital tissue. We often use it as a supplement to testosterone pills, but do not prescribe it for libido problems, which are better treated orally. We've found the cream to be highly effective in increasing genital sensation in women during sexual stimulation and intercourse.

Testosterone cream is available from the same compounding pharmacies as testosterone capsules. The dosage we prefer is 2 percent testosterone in cream form, although it can vary depending on the patient from 1 to 3 percent. It should be applied three times a week at bedtime and half an hour before sex if it doesn't fall on one of those days, in carefully dispensed amounts. Using too much can result in increased genital hair growth or an enlargement of the clitoris. As with testosterone pills, pregnant women and women planning to conceive should not use testosterone cream.

Prostaglandin E-1 cream: Drug companies are currently developing a topical genital cream for both women and men to enhance arousal and orgasm. Prostaglandin E-1 (PGE1) is a factor that relaxes smooth muscle tissue and, like

Viagra, helps to open up the blood vessels. PGE1 is actually used to induce uterine contractions and has been used to induce abortions. Before Viagra, a synthetic form of PGE1, marketed as Caverject, was one of the few treatments for male impotence. It is effective but a little unpleasant in that a man has to administer it to himself by inserting a needle into the side of his penis about 20 minutes before he plans to have intercourse. For now, we don't know how well the topical PGE1 will work in women, but the concept is promising.

Phentolamine: Like sildenafil, phentolamine is a blood-flow enhancing agent, and has been used in penile injections to treat impotence. Phentolamine is now being tested in oral form. The Food and Drug Administration put trials in humans on a temporary clinical hold after a two-year study showed that a small number of rats given phentolamine developed benign tumors called brown fat proliferations. These were found to be benign and the hold was lifted.

Marketed by Zonagen as Vasomax for men and as Vasotem for women, phentolamine is a short-term, alpha-adrenergic receptor blocker. In essence it works by overriding the nerves that block the penis from becoming engorged and erect. It works faster than sildenafil, as quickly as 15 minutes after ingestion, and can be used by people who take nitrate-based heart medicines. A recent study on women in Mexico showed improved sexual arousal.

Apomorphine: Apomorphine was initially used as a treatment for Parkinson's disease. It targets the brain and stimulates the release of dopamine, the brain chemical involved in sensations of pleasure and the erection response. A new apomorphine treatment to be taken in a tablet under the tongue is currently under development by TAP Pharmaceuticals in Lake Forest, Illinois. Called Uprima, this would be the first drug for sexual dysfunction to target the brain, the starting point for sexual arousal. In essence, apomorphine gets involved in the human sexual response at an earlier part of the process than Viagra.

The FDA had been expected to approve Uprima in 2000, but in April of that year an FDA panel raised concerns about its possible side effects, including nausea and vomiting in some patients. In July 2000, TAP withdrew its application for approval in the United States. At this writing, TAP was planning to resubmit its request after collecting additional data from trials that were to conclude at the end of 2000.

Like Vasomax, Uprima works in about 15 minutes. It's safe for people who take nitrate-based heart medications. Its principal drawback is that it causes nausea and vomiting and even fainting in some patients.

L-Arginine and yohimbine: A combination of L-Arginine, an amino acid available over the counter in health food stores, and yohimbine, a powder made from the inner bark of the yohimbine tree of West Africa, is currently being tested. L-Arginine has been around for years as a dietary supplement and vitamin, but recently it has attracted more interest because it is a precursor to the formation of nitric oxide, which we now know is a mediator of sexual response in both men and women. Yohimbine has been around forever as an herbal medicine used to improve libido. Some people say it helps to improve erections in men, but many doctors consider it a placebo that works because men think it will. Yohimbine is an alpha 2 adrenergic blocker that has been used for the treatment of male erectile dysfunction. Results have not been promising in men.

We're interested in seeing how yohimbine works in combination with L-Arginine. The two together are being evaluated for treatment of female sexual arousal disorder in postmenopausal women, and initial results look promising.

The Eros-CTD (clitoral therapy device): In May 2000 this became the first treatment for female sexual dysfunction approved by the FDA. Developed by UroMetrics, Inc., the clitoral therapy device is in essence a small pump with a tiny plastic cup attachment that fits over the clitoris and surrounding tissue. It provides gentle suction, simulating the sucking effects of oral sex and stimulating blood flow to the area. It's not meant to replace a vibrator, but it does cause orgasms in some women. The device might also prevent the fibrosis (collagen deposits) in aging women that build up in the arteries leading to the clitoris. Although some women with sexual arousal complaints like to use the Eros-CTD for the stimulation effects, it may also over time prevent fibrosis of the clitoris that occurs with aging, by enhancing blood flow in the arteries leading to the clitoris. Thus, this device may have a preventive role as well as a therapeutic one.

Nerve-sparing surgery: It was in the early 1980s that Patrick C. Walsh, a urologist, professor, and chair of the Johns Hopkins Brady Urological Institute, developed what is sometimes called the "Walsh procedure," or "nerve-sparing" radical prostatectomy. This is now a standard operation for treatment of prostate cancer that preserves erections in many patients. Before Dr. Walsh's significant contribution, as recently as the 1970s, men were in the same place that women are now. Doctors were ignorant about the precise causes of erectile dysfunction and unaware of the location of the nerves and blood vessels responsible for normal erections.

As Dr. Walsh recounts in his book, *The Prostate: A Guide for Men and the Women Who Love Them*, two things happened. First, new surgical methods in the late 1970s made the operation less bloody and safer. Second, the new "bloodless field," as surgeons called it, enabled them to actually see what they were doing. Dr. Walsh discovered that the microscopic bundles of nerves that run to the spongy, erectile bodies in the penis are actually outside the capsule of the prostate—meaning that a surgeon could get rid of all the cancer but still avoid cutting the nerves. Until then, those nerves had almost always been damaged during surgery, simply because doctors didn't know they existed. Once they did, they learned how to avoid them. As a result of Dr. Walsh's techniques, urologists began cutting more carefully and patients were often able to retain their ability to have an erection. The same is now true for colorectal surgeons who perform rectal resections in men (although nerve-sparing surgery is sometimes precluded in patients with rectal cancer).

In women, we are perhaps at least a half-century behind. Incredibly, we know less about female pelvic anatomy than we did thirty years ago about male genital anatomy. Our goal is to define female pelvic anatomy, in particular the pathways of the important nerves and blood vessels to the genital area. From there we hope to develop similar nerve-sparing pelvic surgeries for women. What we do know is that the nerves and blood vessels important to the genitals originate on the spinal cord. But we don't know with 100-percent certainty their relationship to the uterus, cervix, and vagina. If we knew, we might be able to rethink how we perform hysterectomies and other pelvic surgery. This lack of knowledge is what spurred Jennifer's interest in this field during her residency training. She was also surprised by the fact that her surgeon mentors knew relatively little about female sexual anatomy compared to male anatomy and that few efforts were being made to improve this discrepancy between the sexes.

Jennifer aims to identify these structures and develop special nerve-sparing operations for women. Based on our research so far, we know that there are bundles of nerves and arteries along the sides of the cervix. (See figure 5.2.) The question is what is their precise course from inside the pelvis to the genital structures, and how can we modify surgical techniques to preserve them. One method we are investigating for hysterectomy (for benign disease, not cancer) involves close dissection at the level of the cervix, sparing as much as possible of the uterosacral and cardinal ligaments. Isolation of the uterine artery, by trying to spare the vaginal branches, may also prevent damage.

Treatments for pelvic floor prolapse vary depending on the extent of the problem and the type of symptoms. Today, surgery for incontinence is much less invasive than it was even 10 years ago and is now usually performed as an outpatient procedure. The typical surgery involves the placement of a sling or hammock to support the sagging bladder. Less invasive procedures include injections of collagen as well as a new synthetic material into the urethra to increase resistance and prevent leakage.

Figure 5.2 Nerves and arteries to uterus and vagina, site of injury during surgery

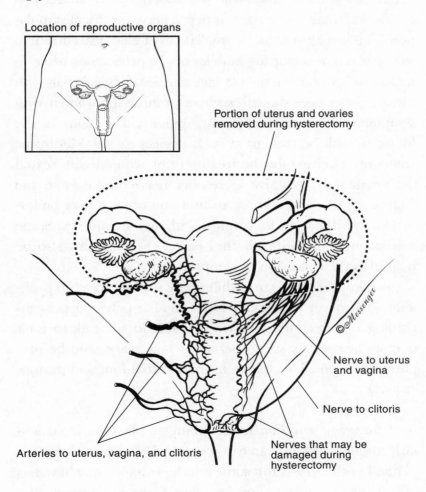

Location of reproductive organs

Portion of uterus and ovaries removed during hysterectomy

Nerve to uterus and vagina

Nerve to clitoris

Arteries to uterus, vagina, and clitoris

Nerves that may be damaged during hysterectomy

Until recently, urologists and gynecologists specializing in pelvic floor problems have focused primarily on restoring normal urinary and bowel anatomy and function. With Dr. Schlomo Raz at UCLA Medical Center, Jennifer hopes to contribute to new surgical techniques to improve or restore sexual function in women who will undergo pelvic surgery.

An alternative to surgery is pelvic nerve electrical stimulation. This involves the use of small doses of electrical current to strengthen the supporting muscles of the pelvic floor while simultaneously relaxing the bladder muscles. Clinical trials with these devices have shown excellent promise for women with symptoms of urinary frequency, urgency, and pain. In the future we will be looking at such devices as the Medtronic Interstim Therapy for the treatment of women with sexual dysfunction as well. By increasing nerve impulses to the vagina, uterus, and clitoris, arousal and orgasm may be improved, particularly in women with nerve injuries. Some medications, biofeedback, and Kegel exercises can also be helpful in the reduction of symptoms.

It is important to stress that many women have no problems whatsoever with sexual function after pelvic surgery, including hysterectomy. But women should still talk to their doctors before any such operations take place, and be prepared for a possible change in their sexual function postoperatively.

Changing medications: Many medications, particularly antidepressants, can cause sexual dysfunction, as we explained in chapter 4. But some antidepressants may have less of an adverse affect, among them Celexa, Serzone, and Wellbutrin. In May 2000, a study led by Dr. R. Taylor Seagraves of the Case Western University School of Medicine found that 15 of 51 women who had little or no sexual desire experienced an increase in desire after taking Wellbutrin. The study was financed by Glaxo Wellcome, Inc., the maker of Wellbutrin. Oral contraceptives may need to be reevaluated as well, either by changing to a lower dose, or in some cases by switching to a different form of contraception.

Women who think their medication may be causing sexual problems should talk to their doctors about switching or changing the dose.

Treatment for other physical problems: Women who have sexual dysfunction caused by heart disease, high blood pressure, high cholesterol, diabetes, smoking, or other physical problems need to address the primary condition first. In some cases, taking care of the primary disease may improve or resolve the sexual problem without further treatment.

Good health: As with many other health problems, sexual problems can be improved with good health habits. Women should exercise regularly, eat a low-fat diet, get enough sleep, drink alcohol only in moderation, and not smoke. (See chapter 8 for the positive effects of exercise on sexual function.) They should also have sex—that's a good habit, too, because it keeps the blood flowing to the genital area. The old adage, "If you don't use it, you'll lose it," may very well be true in the case of sexual function in both men and women.

Therapy

Psychotherapy is the foundation for all successful treatment of sexual dysfunction and will likely remain so. There are two kinds of talk therapy that help with sexual dysfunction. One is sex therapy, which focuses specifically on sexual problems or, in a couple, the sexual relationship. The other is standard psychotherapy, which focuses generally on emotions and relationship problems. When two partners are involved, it's called couples therapy. Counseling, another useful intervention, is usually more of a short-term educational program that provides a woman with information about anatomy, sexual practices, vibrators, other sexual devices, and more. In our clinic, we often end up providing a kind of combination therapy that encompasses all three types.

Sex therapy is simply another form of talk therapy either for couples or an individual. Individual sex therapy is called for when a woman's emotional history or emotional health is affecting her sex life, such as childhood sexual abuse. The problem may cause a woman to feel great shame and anxiety about her sexuality. In sex therapy with couples, the therapist theoretically takes over the couple's sexual relationship to help them redefine it. Intercourse, usually a source of great tension, is temporarily removed from the relationship. The idea is to build the sexual relationship from the ground up, without the pressures or expectations of sexual performance, so the couple can work on and enhance sexual communication and effectively resolve sexual conflict.

As a general routine, a couple meets for an hour of talk on a weekly basis with the therapist, who provides "homework" assignments. Couples are usually asked to start with sensual touching. The idea is to move through the stages of sexual intimacy slowly and consistently, allowing for the couple to build on their sexual communication and techniques along the way. Sex therapy also allows a couple to identify relationship pitfalls that adversely affect their sexuality. (For more on sex therapy, see chapters 6 and 7.)

Often, serious emotional and relationship issues arise,

like problems with resentment, anger, child rearing, intimacy, self-esteem, or major changes in life. These conflicts may push the sex therapy into a more traditional couples therapy. More often than not, treatment involves an interactive combination of general couples therapy and sex therapy.

Janet was only seven years old when she was sexually abused by her 19-year-old brother-in-law, who forced her to perform oral sex on him. The abuse continued until she was 13. By the time she came to see us, she was 35, married, with two children, and was working as a teacher at a Boston nursery school. Although Janet had spoken up about the abuse long ago, and thought her family had supported her, she was beginning to wonder if she was really "OK with it," as she put it to Laura. She was also concerned that the abuse might be at the root of the sexual problems in her marriage.

Janet could reach an orgasm only by self-stimulation, she told us, but she had never been able to have one with her husband, or with anyone else. She would "shut down" right before she seemed to reach orgasm. "My body is shaking," Janet said, "and I stay, stay, stay there. It drives me out of my mind." Her husband had reacted to his wife's problem by withdrawing from sex, and the two were now in marriage counseling. Janet was in tears as she described to Laura the impasse at home: "My husband said to me a little while ago, 'What are we going to do if we can't fix this problem? Live without sex? We can't. We'll have to get a divorce.'"

Laura told Janet that her "shutdown" response might be a kind of automatic reaction that many children use to cope with long-term sexual abuse. In order to survive abuse as it is happening, children tend to "disassociate" themselves, either going blank in their minds or sometimes imagining pleasant fantasylands that take them away from the horror of where they are. It's an important survival skill at that time, but it can extend unintentionally into adult life. In Janet's case, it affected the way she experienced her sexuality. In order to survive the abuse, Janet had shut off all awareness and emotions connected to the abuse. However, in adulthood, she was still disassociating during sexual activity, even with her own husband.

Janet wanted to try Viagra, and she did several times, with little response. We weren't surprised. Sildenafil works best when there are primary physiological problems, not emotional ones. But the Viagra did convince Janet that what she needed to do was to explore her feelings about the abuse, her relationship with her husband, and her sexuality. Laura warned her that it would most likely be extraordinarily painful to start talking openly about her abuse history. She might have to revisit the trauma and move through it emotionally, much as if she were experiencing the death of a loved one again. Janet said she was ready.

As Janet began seeing Laura regularly for psychotherapy, her feelings exploded. "Oh, my God," she told Laura soon after their sessions began. "I had no idea how messed up I was." As time went on, Janet became angry with her family for what she came to see as their inadequate response. Although they had believed her and made sure she received counseling, they hadn't pressed charges against the brother-in-law, or even told the rest of the family. Janet continued to have to see him at family events. She was particularly angry with her sister, even though her sister had divorced her abusive husband years before.

Janet told her other siblings, who hadn't known before,

what had happened. They were supportive, but talking about the abuse with them brought more memories to the surface and forced her to remember more details. She became deeply depressed, unable to sleep or control her crying. At one point, she told Laura that she hadn't been able to get thoughts of her niece with a penis in her mouth out of her head. "There was nothing that would make it stop," she said. "It was just pounding, pounding, pounding." The emotional pain became so overwhelming that Janet began to fantasize about her own death, what we call suicidal ideation. Laura didn't think that Janet was at high risk for taking her own life, because Janet had no plan for carrying out a suicide, and felt very clear that she would never act on her fantasy. Still, Laura closely monitored her.

Antianxiety and antidepressant medication helped, and after a few months, as September and the start of the school year neared, Janet began to improve. She told Laura that she thought she had almost "allowed" herself to have her crisis in the slower, summer months.

Still, Janet's sex life, not surprisingly, was now nonexistent. As she continued to heal, she and her husband, who had been supportive throughout her crisis, decided they needed to start over again. Today, Janet believes the abuse is not past her—"It's a process that I think is going to take years," she told Laura—but she feels healthy enough to work on her marriage. She and her husband began sex therapy with Laura, and treatment will be focused on helping Janet reclaim her sexual life on her terms.

People often ask if sex therapy really works. It does, but a couple has to be engaged and committed, and have a good relationship with a skilled sex therapist.

Drugs to treat sexual dysfunction, like sildenafil and

testosterone, have made the job of the sex therapist much easier. Much of our work in the past was focused on the grieving over the loss of sexual function that we now know may be medically based. Today, as we are better able to tend to the physical problems, sex therapy is more successful.

CHAPTER SIX

Sexuality through the Life Cycle

A woman's sexuality is a journey, always changing, never static. Sexual desires and responses ebb and flow, shifting with adolescence, young adulthood, marriage or life with a partner, pregnancy, child rearing, menopause, and aging. Sexuality is always there, in one form or another. Children, in fact, are sexual from birth.

In this chapter we'll examine what a woman can expect as she makes her sexual journey through life. In order for a woman to understand how her early childhood and adolescent experiences, in particular the attitudes of her parents, have affected her sexuality, she must consider where and how sexual problems may have developed. Aline Zolbrod, in her book, *Sex Smart: How Your Childhood Shaped Your Sexual Life and What to Do about It*, focuses on how early childhood experiences shape the way adults experience their sexual lives and discusses ways of addressing these conflicts. We feel it is important that women understand what to expect in terms of the sexual changes that occur throughout their lives and the reasons for these changes.

Childhood

Sexuality in the period that stretches from birth through preadolescence was once seen as nonexistent, and if it existed in any form, it was considered inappropriate or even dangerous. We now know that sexual feelings in children are normal and healthy, and that a warm, secure, and physically affectionate relationship between a primary caretaker and a child is not sexual, but rather essential to a child's ability to form loving relationships as an adult. Babies adore cuddling, and although they're too young to understand the connections to their future sexual lives, they do know that physical closeness feels good.

Masturbation can start as soon as a child discovers his or her genitals. One mother reported that the first time her toddler boy sat in the bath and noticed his genitals, he reached down to grab them, thinking they were another bath toy, but jerked back in surprise because he'd grabbed quite hard. But children learn very quickly that touching their genitals is pleasurable and will naturally tend to continue these "feel good" behaviors. Most children play with their genitals simply because the experience is pleasurable and relaxing. There are even documented cases of children having what seem to be orgasms as early as six months (this occurs without ejaculation in boys because the testicles do not produce sperm or seminal fluid until puberty). It's clear from the described physical symptoms of heavy breathing and reflex pelvic thrusting during genital stimulation against a pillow or stuffed toy, for instance, that they're doing what feels good.

Unfortunately, many of our patients were taught from an early age that their genital area was dirty and touching themselves was wrong or even sinful. Many had their hands angrily slapped or pushed away from their genitals and were made to feel ashamed and guilty about their sexual feelings. A child easily internalizes those negative feelings about sex, which can play out in later life, as we see too often in our patients. A woman whose mother told her repeatedly as a child that masturbation and the resulting pleasurable feelings were sinful may have difficulty letting go sexually as an adult. In some cases, she may also feel embarrassed about her naked body and ashamed of her sexual feelings.

Parents shouldn't be alarmed about children displaying sexual feelings. When children see parents naked, they'll invariably point and ask, "What's that?" Parents should tell them, using the correct words, like vagina, penis, breasts, and anus. Negative slang can give the impression that there is something shameful about those body parts. The next question is often, "Can I touch it?" Here the response should be "No, that belongs to mommy or daddy, just like your penis or vulva belongs to you."

This is a good time to tell children about inappropriate touching—in other words, your body is yours, you control it, and no one should be allowed to touch you in ways you don't want. If that happens, a child should be instructed to tell her parents or another trusted caretaker. At the same time, a child should be told that another adult should never tell her secrets, or do things to her, that she can't tell her parents. Children should be encouraged to feel safe sharing anything with their parents. This will help protect your children in the future, and set the stage for later talks about safe sex, AIDS, and other concerns of adolescence. As we saw in Janet's case in chapter 5, a child who suppresses her concerns or abuse suffers for it as an adult.

When children ask about where babies come from, answer their questions directly and matter-of-factly. But you don't need to tell them everything at a very young age. When they ask more specifically, usually around the ages of 9 or 10, although it varies widely, be sure to provide them with more than the basic biological information. Children need to understand that sex is an emotional and pleasurable experience, and they need to know the values you attach to it. Be sure to tell both boys and girls about menstruation and sexual responses, and be sure to include AIDS, other sexually transmitted diseases, prostitution, and sexual abuse. Children will hear about these topics at school or on television, and it's important that they learn the facts first, and correctly, from you. Many adults today would have avoided sexual problems if their parents had been open with them about these issues.

Parents should also tell their children about sexual orientation. Although the appropriate time varies with each child, most children by the later elementary school years have heard about homosexuals, and it's important to pass on accurate information that reflects your values. Although most children aren't aware of their own sexual orientation until they reach the teen years, some feel different from others of their gender at a very young age.

With all the sexual information you provide to your children, we stress that information does not mean permission. Study after study shows that the more information children have about sex, the wiser the decisions they make later in life.

Adolescence

Adolescence is the transition period from childhood to adulthood, and is marked by the physical changes, mood swings, and self-consciousness that are the hallmarks of puberty. Puberty, the transformation from sexual immaturity to maturity usually begins anywhere from the ages of 8 to 13 and extends into the late teens. Most girls enter puberty at around the same time that their mothers did, but many girls these days are beginning much earlier. Doctors are now readjusting the standards that exist in many current medical textbooks, which say that only 1 percent of girls younger than 8 show signs of puberty.

In 1999 in the journal *Pediatrics*, for example, Dr. Paul B. Kaplowitz, Dr. Sharon E. Oberfield, and members of the Lawson Wilkins Pediatric Endocrine Society concluded that the onset of breast development was noted in American white girls as young as 7 and in African-American girls as young as 6. Doctors can't yet explain this earlier onset of puberty, but speculate that it might be caused by better nutrition, fewer diseases, childhood obesity, hormones present in beef and milk, or exposure to insecticides. In any case, the age of menarche, a girl's first menstrual period, has declined steadily in the United States over the last century. In 1890, the average age of menarche in the United States was nearly 15. Today it's not quite 12½, according to a 1997 study in *Pediatrics* of 17,000 girls.

Puberty begins in girls when three important glands of the endocrine system—the hypothalamus, the pituitary gland, and the ovaries—begin to produce hormones. The endocrine system is the name for the network of glands and glandular tissue that secretes hormones into the body. The hypothalamus is the portion of the brain that has the primary control over the endocrine system. The pituitary is an acorn-sized gland at the base of the brain. The ovaries in the pelvis secrete both estrogen and testosterone.

Breast buds develop first, as early as ages 6 or 7, as we have discussed, but typically anywhere from ages 8 to 11. Many girls also experience a growth spurt in height and weight at this time. Pubic hair appears, followed about a year later by underarm hair and an increase in the amount of sweat produced by the glands under the arms. The labia, or genital lips, enlarge, as do the vagina and uterus. Body fat accumulates on the hips and buttocks, giving a girl the beginning of womanly curves. Testosterone increases oil production in the skin pores, which can cause acne. Mood swings, embarrassment, and self-consciousness about the body are common, and normal, at this age.

Menstruation usually begins between the ages of 11 and 14 in developed countries and is often preceded for 6 months to a year by a white vaginal discharge, made up of secretions from the vaginal walls. Although menstrual periods may be irregular for the first few years because ovulation doesn't always occur, a girl can get pregnant as soon as she begins menstruating.

This is also a crucial time in the development of sexual identity and orientation. Although some reports have indicated that it is more common for boys to experiment with homosexuality in adolescence, girls do, too. But there may still be a great deal of guilt attached to the experience, especially among girls whose families have negative attitudes toward homosexuality. Unfortunately, girls and boys who suspect they are homosexual are far more likely than other children to suffer from depression, to abuse drugs and alcohol, and to attempt suicide. In fact, almost 30 percent of teenage suicides in the United States are committed by homosexual youths. The fortunate girls and boys are the ones who were made to feel comfortable with their sexual orientation and were able to talk to their parents about their questions or fears. Most important, they were reassured that their sexual orientation has nothing to do with their parents' love.

Whether girls grow up as homosexuals or heterosexuals, they are intensely aware at this stage of their own sexual feelings. A girl might notice a tingling in her genitals when she sees something that arouses her, like a romantic movie, or she might become aroused at an erotic thought. It's a distinct departure from the sexuality she experienced as a child, when it was focused on how she felt about her body. Now sexuality begins to be connected to her feelings about others.

Although girls may have sex as early as 12 or perhaps even earlier, more typically at this stage there is a great deal of preliminary, noninsertive, "practice" sexual activity at this age—kissing, petting, hours spent staring into a romantic partner's face. By the time a girl is 15 or 16, she often has a great deal of sexual desire, but no way of knowing how to translate it into acceptable or appropriate action. Sex education is crucial at this age, as well as information about birth control options and the risks of pregnancy, HIV, and other sexually transmitted diseases. We've found that girls who were provided with this kind of help felt more comfortable with their own sexuality as adults. And rather than encouraging them to have sex, the open approach empowered them to do just the opposite and say "no" until they were ready. We suggest that parents of teenagers encourage open communication and try to have discussions about relationships and sexuality. Although teenagers often withdraw from their parents at this stage in their development and feel that such open discussions are more like "lectures," they need to feel that the lines of communication are open if needed or desired.

In the United States in 1995, half of girls between the ages of 15 to 19 had had sexual intercourse, which is actually a slight decline from earlier years. The statistics come from the National Survey of Family Growth, a federal study conducted among more than 10,000 women by the United States Department of Health and Human Services. In 1990 the department found that 55 percent of girls between the ages of 15 and 19 had had sexual intercourse. Perhaps more telling is that in the 1995 survey nearly a quarter of teenage girls who had sex described their first sexual intercourse as "voluntary but not wanted"—meaning that they may have been pressured by boyfriends, peers, or social expectations.

At this stage, girls are often confused about when and if they are ready to be sexual. Girls should decide for themselves, but it's often hard to know whether they genuinely want to have sex, or just want to please a partner. A girl should ask herself how committed she is to the relationship, and why she feels she wants to have sex; for instance, because she is in love, because she feels left out from her other friends who have had sex, or because she is curious. Asking these questions helps a young girl or boy make an informed decision. If a girl does have intercourse at this stage, she is better off emotionally if she is practicing safe sex and is close to her partner. Some girls are able to talk to their parents about their experiences, but many are not. Most feel guilty about having to lie to their parents, which does nothing to help their comfort level with a sexual relationship.

Some girls at this age learn to self-stimulate as a healthy,

safe way of relieving the powerful sexual tension of adolescence. It also teaches girls that there are more ways to be sexual than just having intercourse. Self-stimulation helps to
make girls more comfortable with their own bodies and helps
lay the groundwork for a positive self-image. It also makes a
girl aware of her body and how it responds, which invariably
will help her to achieve sexual fulfillment. And just because a
girl self-stimulates doesn't mean she's going to run out and
have sex. It may actually have the opposite effect.

In our practice, many of our patients had their first sexual intercourse experience around the age of 15 or 16. Every
single one remembers it quite well, of course, but Laura can
count on one hand the number of patients who say they enjoyed the experience and fewer still who had an orgasm. In
her book *The First Time: What Parents and Teenage Girls Should
Know about Losing Your Virginity*, Karen Bouris reports similar
findings when she interviewed 150 American women 20 to 70
years of age about their first experience with intercourse.
Only a minimal number said that their first time was a positive experience, and even fewer said that they had reached
orgasm. Orgasm isn't necessarily the goal, but it does tell
you how many women were perhaps not ready for sex. Still,
many say they did enjoy the experience in other ways—the
physical closeness, for example, or the feelings of emotional
intimacy. We've also found that the older a woman is at the
time of her first sexual experience, the more she may enjoy
it. A woman who waits to have sex tends to be more of a full
partner in the experience. A younger girl is more apt to take
her cues from a partner who is usually not much more sexually educated than she is.

Plenty of women do make mistakes when they're young.
They drink too much at a party, for example, and have sex

with someone they do not know very well and who they may never see again. Adolescence is a time to make mistakes and learn from them. Most women recover just fine. For others, particularly women with low self-esteem and women who were taught that sex is dirty or wrong, the first sexual experience can be devastating and may affect later sexuality.

One of our patients, Jill, had her first sexual experience in her teens with a boyfriend who later rejected her, saying that she wasn't a good lover. When Jill came to see us, she was 25 and a production coordinator for a Web site. By then she realized that the boyfriend hadn't been a good lover himself. Her problem today is lack of libido.

Although she had been with her current boyfriend, Mike, for five years and was very committed to him, "I've never felt very confident," she told Laura during their first session. She related her experience with her first boyfriend: "He was a quick lover, I'll tell you that. I wasn't very responsive, but it was mostly because I didn't know what to do. I don't think he knew what to do either." After the boyfriend broke up with her, Jill was devastated. To make matters worse, he would call to tell her about the great sex he was having with other women. (He clearly had issues of his own.)

By the time Jill got to college, she was having highly satisfying sex with another boyfriend. Then she met Mike, and the couple quickly became close. The sex with him, Jill said, was terrific, at least for the first year and a half. But into the second year of the relationship, once she began to let down her emotional guard, she became extremely anxious and suffered from an episode of depression. She felt the depression and anxiety developed in part due to her obsession with Mike's past girlfriends and his prior sexual relationships with them. These thoughts consumed her and she began to feel sexually inadequate. Jill's anxiety and depression could also have been related in part to her having just left home to go to college and adjusting to a new world of relationships and academic demands. Without the supportive cocoon of home, these new pressures can lead to anxiety and depression in young adults.

In Jill's case, by the time she recovered from the depression, her sexual desire had significantly waned. When she came to see us, she was taking no antidepressants, so her problems could not have been related to medications. Her desire continued to decline over time, creating enormous tension in the relationship. When she came to see us, at first on her own, she and Mike hadn't had sex in a year.

"It's been very, very tough," she said. "I just don't feel normal. I go through life feeling like I'm set apart from everyone else. I meet couples and I think about them having sex, and I'm very aware that I'm not having it. I always assume that everyone is having fantastic sex. I'm just so sure of it."

Jill's despair was very much her own, but it is something we hear often from other patients. Almost every woman who comes into our office talks about how incomplete she feels as a result of her sexual dysfunction, even when she is treated like a sexual object by others. Inside she feels that she's not quite right, that she has to carry on with the facade. This can be devastating in many cases. Most women have told very few people about their problems. They feel shame, as if they are inadequate as women, which worsens their feelings of failure.

Jill's issues seemed to be more emotional than physical, and she wasn't particularly interested in undergoing our standard medical and physiologic evaluation. (See chapter 1.) Laura began seeing her for therapy, and quickly found Jill to be an intelligent, articulate, and very self-aware young woman. "I've had a lot of betrayals with boyfriends," Jill said. "I've built up a little wall in the last few years. I haven't told people about this problem, but I have this huge interior monologue, and part of me likes it that way." She also seemed to understand that her first sexual experience, however painful, was not the sole cause of her problem.

"It's one of the accessories of the problem," she said. "It's just a contributing factor. It planted a little seed that grew. I think the root of the problem is that I'm ambivalent about commitment." These feelings were made worse by the fact that Mike was somewhat withdrawn emotionally. "I'm a closed person," he said. "I like to establish boundaries." Still, Jill said that she was devoted to Mike. Even though their sexual life was troubled, she felt that the relationship was solid at its core, and worth trying to save. "I guess that's the cruel irony of it," she said. "Even when things were bad, we were still having a very good time."

Laura suggested that Mike come in for counseling with Jill, which he did willingly. The two engaged in a combination of couples and sex therapy. They met with Laura for one 50-minute session per week, during which Laura gave them assignments in the form of sexual exercises to work on at home. As is standard with sex therapy, Laura first asked them to remove sexual intercourse—or, in their case, all the worrying about not having sexual intercourse—from the relationship. She then asked them to start from the beginning with gentle sensual touching, cuddling, and massage. Each week, as long as all was going well, Laura gave them assignments that moved them gradually closer to sexual intercourse, including "imitating" intercourse; that is, Laura asked them to get into the position for intercourse and engage in genital touching but not penetration during their at-home exercises.

As the exercises progressed, Jill and Mike "processed" them, meaning that they discussed their reactions and feelings to the sexual and nonsexual exercises and to each other in the talk sessions with Laura. They also worked on their general communication skills. Mike eventually came to the point where he didn't blame Jill for their sexual difficulties but rather began to acknowledge the role he played in their problems. The two ended up communicating better, fighting less, and feeling more connected. As a result, Jill felt that much of the tension the couple had once experienced was now removed. "We're less nervous each time," she said in the course of the treatment. "And we talk about it afterward. That helps." Jill found her sexual response to be good once she began the exercises, and was at times aroused to the point of needing to masturbate after a session. (Although couples in sex therapy are asked to refrain from intercourse until the therapist permits it, they are allowed to self-stimulate in private, and then together, if they wish, in later stages of therapy.)

For Jill, the vulnerability she experienced in her sexual relationships was anxiety producing and may also have been a defensive mechanism to keep a relationship at bay. In order to be sexual, you have to be willing to allow yourself to be vulnerable with someone else, to let that person in emotionally. That doesn't mean Jill wasn't in love with Mike, but it does mean that she may have had unresolved issues about intimacy and control. She and Laura continued to work on those. As for that first sexual experience, Jill was right when she described it as one of the "accessories" to the problem. But as is often the case, early sexual experiences set the stage for the way we experience sexuality later in life.

One early sexual experience that can have a devastating affect on adult sexuality is sexual abuse. In the United States, studies show that nearly one in four women has experienced some form of sexual abuse. In a 1992 study in Washington state by the Alan Guttmacher Institute, 23 percent of 3,128 girls in eighth, tenth, and twelfth grades reported that they had been sexually abused. There have been similar results in other countries: in a 1997 study published in the *Medical Journal of Australia*, one in five of the 710 Australian women surveyed reported suffering sexual abuse during childhood.

In our practice, nearly 30 percent of our patients have suffered some form of sexual abuse. Abuse ranges from unwanted fondling to oral sex and rape, but it also includes, for instance, being forced to look at pornography or being forced to listen to "dirty" talk. If a young girl's first sexual experience is abusive, it harms or destroys not only her trust and self-esteem but also her developing sexual identity. Women who have been abused may feel shame, isolation, and guilt. They may blame themselves, particularly if they became aroused during the abuse, or if they become involved in long-term relationships with their abusers. They may turn what should be anger toward the abuser inward— toward themselves—which typically manifests itself as depression. Studies have linked sexual abuse to posttraumatic stress disorder, eating disorders, gastrointestinal problems, and higher risks of suicide.

As with Janet, the woman who was repeatedly molested

by her brother-in-law as a child (see chapter 5), abuse victims often have enormous trouble in their later sexual relationships. Janet disassociated during sex with her husband and shut down just before reaching orgasm. The act of disassociating the sexual experience, of "going somewhere else" in one's mind, is a coping mechanism that abused children typically use to take themselves emotionally away from the terrible things that are happening to them. Janet was able to become aroused but never felt "the release" either alone or with her partner.

But it's important to say here that childhood sexual abuse is not a sentence to lifelong sexual dysfunction. Women with abuse histories can reach a level of resolution. Obviously, the less traumatic the abuse, the more likely it is that a woman can sustain healthy sexual relationships as an adult. Much depends on the nature of the abuse and how it was handled, especially by primary caregivers. Recovery is very different, for example, for a woman who was raped repeatedly by her father and told no one than it is for a woman who was molested once by a neighbor's visiting cousin, told her supportive parents, and then pressed charges.

Counseling is crucial. The first step is acknowledging what happened, the second is acknowledging that it wasn't your fault, and the third is purging the shame. Mourning, letting the pain go, and getting angry at the perpetrator are all very liberating, and essential to recovery.

Young Adulthood

By the late teens and early twenties, the hormones of adolescence have quieted and the physical changes have slowed.

Most women have stopped growing. Their menstrual periods and moods have become more predictable. This is a time of new freedom but also pressures as young people find jobs, gain some economic independence, and begin living on their own. Many women, their libidos strong, suddenly find themselves facing more sexual freedom than they ever had before, which is both exhilarating and frightening. It is an important time to practice safer sex. The rituals of dating can be bewildering: At what point in a relationship do you have sex? In big American cities, among young professionals, many young men and women report that the pivotal moment seems to be the third date, the point at which a relationship either becomes intimate or not. Women need to know that if this is too fast for them—and it is, for many, many women—they can tell their partners that they're not ready, that they need more time. Empowerment is as much about advocating for your sexual needs as it is about declining unwanted sexual advances.

During the pre-AIDS, post–birth control pill era of the 1960s and 1970s, sexuality was looser and sexual experimentation more prevalent. But the spread of sexually transmitted diseases now means that women at this stage must talk to their partners about their sexual histories and negotiate for safer sex—laying down the rule, for example, that there will be no intercourse without a condom. All of this requires open communication. The time to have sex is not necessarily on the third date, but when a woman can communicate her sexual—and safer sexual—needs to her partner, and feel comfortable with the level of emotional and physical intimacy.

For young adults, one of the greatest psychosocial tasks is separating from the family and finding a way in the world as a grown-up. The freedom exponentially increases while the judgment may not. Therefore, many young women may find themselves in precarious positions, such as drinking too much at a party and finding themselves in a date rape situation or getting involved in sexual relationships with people they would have otherwise avoided with the "excuse" of parental controls.

Furthermore, it can be frightening and lonely making the shift from home to college or to the "real world," particularly at a time when the need for company, security, and reliability are great. Unfortunately, many young men and women seek out relationships that may not be in their best emotional interest.

Historically, young adulthood was the time when women were supposed to find husbands. A good number of older women (many of whom have already entered the ranks of the divorced) joke that they went to college to get an MRS degree, not a BA. The pressure was tremendous to find a husband and if a college girl wasn't "pinned" (one step prior to being engaged) before senior year, she was thought to be a spinster.

Although this has changed tremendously, for many young women the emotional pressure to find Mr. Right continues. Many women still rush into emotional relationships with people to whom they are not well suited. But overall, the generation spawned from the women's movement is a generation of women with careers and lives of their own who can financially afford to take their time in a way that their mothers may not have been able to do.

Married/Couples Life

Most Americans eventually settle down into long-term relationships, married or otherwise. Marriage often causes a profound change in a relationship, even among people who lived together first. For many people, it has a positive effect. A couple can feel connected, liberated, and safe, with more freedom to experiment with sex and take emotional risks. Many surveys show that married people have better sex and feel better about their sexual lives than singles. One study of the sexual practices of nearly 3,500 American men and women, published in 1994 as the book *Sex in America,* found that three-quarters of the married women surveyed said they usually or always had an orgasm during sexual intercourse, compared to 62 percent of single women. The study also found that the married couples had sex more often than singles. (Later, the study was rightfully criticized for its methodology, particularly interviewers who questioned men and women about marital infidelity in front of their spouses. Why would they ever have told the truth?) Still, we think the findings are essentially correct that married women overall are sexually more satisfied with their lives than singles. More specifically, we think it is women in long-term healthy, loving relationships who tend to be more satisfied with their sex lives than singles. Certainly such women tend to have fewer problems with vulnerability and anxiety in sexual relationships. And although the challenge with sex in long-term relationships is to avoid complacency and boredom, the core of trust often allows people to build on their fantasies and expand the sexual relationship.

It's impossible for us to say what is a "normal" amount of

sex in a relationship, even though we're always asked. The insurance companies cover eight to ten Viagra pills per month for men, so that's one judgment on what "normal" frequency is. As another gauge, *Sex in America* found that two-thirds of the respondents, married and single, said they had sex a few times a month or less. From our point of view, the only thing that matters is whether frequency of sex becomes an issue, and whether the desires of the sexual partners are compatible. In other words, if one partner wants to have sex a lot more often than the other, problems can develop. (See chapter 7.) In terms of frequency of intercourse during marriage, each couple sets their own norm, so what other couples are doing should have little relevance. The ups and downs of financial stresses, illness, death of a family member, and raising children affect our personal and sexual relationships. Communication and trust are the keys to working through these stressful issues and maintaining intimacy.

People sometimes ask us to define sexual norms in a relationship—that is, is monogamy realistic and can "open marriage" ever work? Monogamy puts different demands on people who live twice as long today as they did hundreds of years ago, and who may soon consider middle age to start at 65. Many researchers believe that we are evolutionarily conditioned to be serially monogamous. Dr. Helen Fisher, the acclaimed Rutgers University anthropologist, maintains in her book, *Anatomy of Love*, that, like other species, human couples are designed to stay together just long enough to raise a single dependent child through infancy. In the case of humans, about four years. Dr. Fisher also believes that people are built to love more than one person at a time—capable, in other words, of feeling long-term attachment while feeling attracted to someone at the office or on the street.

"Open" relationships are not nearly as socially accepted today as they were in the 1960s and 1970s, at the peak of the sexual revolution. But they do work for some couples, provided there's a tremendous amount of trust and commitment. Many couples who engage in open relationships say they have as close a commitment to each other as monogamous couples. They say they're connected by their hearts and souls, and that their sexuality is just a separate piece that they share with others as well as each other. Open marriage is based on mutual consent and an agreed-upon philosophy and is not the same as infidelity, which is based on betrayal. The downside of open marriage, of course, is that if the trust isn't in place, such a relationship can wreck a marriage.

One final thought: Some couples who have sexual problems prior to marriage think that the marriage will solve them. They want to attribute the problems to something outside the relationship and convince themselves that the troubles will disappear after the wedding. In our experience, this never happens. It is important to seek help for sexual problems long before the honeymoon, or before having a child as an attempt to help save a marriage or resolve marital discord.

Pregnancy and Childbirth

Every woman is different, but the most typical experience that women report during pregnancy is that sexual interest and response in the first and third trimesters is not particularly good but sex in the second trimester is more satisfactory. While this is in fact the experience of many women, no one should ever feel the need to be a sexual athlete during the second three months of pregnancy. There is a certain amount of pressure now with the belief that all women should be swinging from the chandeliers during the second trimester, but it's not necessarily the case.

In the first trimester, many women are often too nauseated and exhausted to be interested in sex. Their breasts may also be very tender and sore. By the second trimester, the nausea usually vanishes as many women report a "surge" of energy. At the same time, hormones have caused the vaginal lips to slightly engorge and have increased vaginal lubrication. Some women feel as if they are constantly in a state of mild sexual arousal. The pressure of the growing baby on the genitals may also cause sensations of genital arousal.

By the last three months, a woman may feel far too cumbersome for sex. Couples who are sexual during these months may need to experiment with new positions, either side-to-side, rear entry, or sitting. A woman may also be worried, unnecessarily in normal pregnancies, that intercourse will harm the baby. Some couples do try intercourse very late in pregnancy as a means of starting labor, but there is no guarantee that it will work, although there is scientific evidence that the prostaglandin in seminal fluid, as well contractions during orgasm, can induce labor.

After delivery, many women feel like strangers in their own bodies, which seem to be oozing fluids from every orifice. It often takes months to feel ready for sex again, particularly if a woman has had a difficult, traumatic delivery that required forceps, suction, or a C-section. An episiotomy, a cut the doctor makes from the base of the vagina toward the anus to make it easier to deliver the baby's head, may cause sexual problems, too. Episiotomy stitches may take four months to heal. A woman's partner should treat her very carefully at first, and understand that intercourse the first time after delivery needs to be gentle. There is now a movement to minimize the need for episiotomies through prenatal training, exercise, and conditioning. In New York City, Maternal Fitness—a program created by Julie Tupler, who wrote a book by the same name—is taught by registered nurses who are also personal trainers and are at the forefront of this trend. (See the Resources section in chapter 9.) The belief is that letting the vagina stretch naturally to allow for the baby's head to pass causes less damage, but this concept is controversial.

Doctors usually tell women to wait six weeks after giving birth before having intercourse again, but when the day comes around, it's important that a woman not feel pressured to have sex if she's not up to it. Some women are, many women aren't. Very often a woman's interest in sex depends on the amount of child-care support she has, and how much she's been able to sleep while caring for a newborn who may well be up three or more times a night.

If a woman had a prolonged labor, the pushing required to get the baby out may have stretched her pelvic floor muscles. Initially she may feel less friction during intercourse, and perhaps less stimulation of her G-spot. This can affect the quality of sexual arousal and orgasms in the weeks after pregnancy, although it is usually temporary. The vagina does shrink back to its normal state within several months, although it may feel larger and looser when a couple first starts to have sex. Kegel exercises can help. (See chapter 9.)

In women who had traumatic deliveries, injury may occur to the pudendal nerve, which provides sensation to the lower third of the vagina and the clitoris. If this occurs, women may experience symptoms ranging from pain to complete loss of sensation. If you experience these symptoms and they persist for more than a few weeks or months, you should speak to your doctor and consider being evaluated by a neurologist.

We have also had a number of patients who have complaints of low libido and have low testosterone levels several years after pregnancy. There are no other descriptions of this "syndrome" in the medical literature, but we believe that many women experience a loss of libido postpartum due to testosterone deficiency. We don't have a biological explanation for why this happens, but we are working on trying to understand what is causing the drop in testosterone in premenopausal women postpartum.

Still, interest in sex after childbirth is not just a matter of overcoming physical complaints. A woman's life has profoundly changed. If it's the first child, she has gone from being part of a pair to part of a triangle, with a demanding baby who takes attention away from the earlier, exclusive relationship. Many women wonder in the days after birth how they will be able to think of themselves as sexual beings again now that their bodies have been so powerfully taken over by motherhood.

Women are also at risk for postpartum depression. Women with a history of depression, or who have depression in their families, are at greater risk. Depression may be chemically induced by the drop in hormones after delivery, which has a tremendous affect on libido. Symptoms include crying, a feeling of sadness, a loss of appetite, lethargy, and sometimes thoughts of suicide or of hurting the baby. Any woman who worries she may be at risk should talk to her doctor about it before delivery so that she can be prepared if the need arises. Many women find it helpful to start building a relationship with a counselor or therapist who specializes in this area while still pregnant.

Breast feeding has different effects on women. Because it causes the release of the hormone oxytocin, which leads to uterine contractions, it is an enormously pleasurable experience for some women. Some women become sexually aroused during breast feeding, and a few have reported having orgasms. It's not that they're sexually aroused by their babies, but such feelings may disturb or confuse them. From our point of view, breast feeding is just serving its evolutionary purpose—if it feels good, you'll be more inclined to keep doing it, and your baby will get the nutrition she needs. Other women find breast feeding more a relaxing than a sexual experience. Since it does use up a significant amount of calories and energy, it puts many women to sleep at a time when they desperately need it.

Breast feeding can also affect sex with a partner. Some women feel that their breasts are suddenly working objects, meant as food for the baby but not pleasure for their partners. It is also common for women to have lubrication problems, since breast feeding can suppress ovulation and the production of estrogen. Other women find the new size, spurting milk, and sensitivity of their breasts highly erotic.

Parenthood

We all know that children as infants are exhausting, and that they can run roughshod over a marriage and intimacy. As they grow older, children may demand less time, but they create new issues for parents' sexual lives.

Laura has had to work with a number of couples simply to make sure that they keep locks on their bedroom doors. It seems a simple device to ensure a fair measure of privacy, but many couples are anxious about the messages they're sending their children. They won't have sex while the children are awake, even though teenagers are up very late with homework or other pursuits. They worry that the children will know they are having sex even though it is a private act for the parents themselves. Many parents don't realize the gift they give their children by allowing themselves to be seen as a loving couple. Children have to get a sense that their parents are their own entity, with space that needs to be respected, and that parents value the relationship enough to take private time for each other. If children see that you're comfortable with your sexuality, that's a good model for them.

Time and again, couples feel that to be good parents they have to put their own relationship aside in order to focus on raising their children. Bringing children into bed with you, a growing trend, doesn't help. Couples sometimes tell Laura that they haven't been on a trip together, or even out on a "date," since the children were born, even years later. If you're truly anxious about baby-sitting, or can't afford it, put the children to bed, go out on the porch, have a glass of wine, and talk. Make sure that the children understand that that's your time together. Ideally, every couple should have a date at least one night a week. There should be no discussion about children or Pampers or daily logistics. It should be a time to share thoughts with each other as two adults. A marriage needs to be tended, just like a new relationship, but far too many couples make it their last priority.

Middle Age and Menopause

The definition of middle age is shifting in America, but we can generally define it as the long period past young adulthood, roughly from ages 40 to 65. In women, physical changes in middle age start with perimenopause, the period of transition into menopause itself, when the body's production of estrogen and testosterone begins to slow. All women are different, but perimenopause generally starts with irregular periods, either heavier or lighter than normal. Menopause, the cessation of a woman's menstrual periods, occurs on average at age 51, and usually lasts several years. (See chapter 4 for a medical description of menopause.) Common symptoms of menopause are hot flashes, vaginal dryness or irritation, incontinence, a thinning or loss of elasticity in the skin, mood swings, and depression. Psychologically, some menopausal women will experience a sense of loss about their childbearing years coming to an end. Some may regret parenting decisions they've made, or simply feel a loss that they will no longer be able to have children of their own.

As with men when they reach middle age, women at the end of their reproductive years often want to take stock of their lives and address the feelings they have about their life choices, the regrets as well as the joys. Menopause can be a wonderful time for many women. They no longer have to worry about pregnancy or child care; they may be nearing retirement, and they can take on new hobbies and interests and build on their relationships.

It's very common for women to have sexual complaints after menopause. The falloff in estrogen and testosterone can cause both a lack of libido and a lack of vaginal lubrication. Blood flow to and sensation in the genital area decrease with age as well, meaning that a woman may have difficulty feeling aroused. She may have less intense orgasms, or they may stop altogether.

Many of the menopausal women who come to see us have been given the message that their drop in libido and diminished sexual sensation are natural parts of aging. But they don't have to be. In addition to hormone replacement therapy, many new medications are being tested, including testosterone and sildenafil, to help the sexual function complaints of menopausal and postmenopausal women. Menopause is not something you have to endure. What's exciting is that the generation of American women now entering menopause is the same generation of women who advocated that more attention be paid to women's sexual health in the 1960s. They don't want to lose their sexuality, nor should they be expected to.

Of course, some women do find that sex no longer carries the same importance and so don't want to receive treatment or take hormones. Others find menopause an enormous relief, or a fresh start, and look upon it as liberation from forty years of worrying about pregnancy

The Golden Years, or Sex after 60

Your body has adjusted to menopause, and it can now truly enter a golden age. Couples no longer have the pressures of child rearing and the financial responsibilities of educating children. They may retire or find a new sense of freedom in traveling. They may go back to school, or change careers. It can be a carefree time, like a honeymoon, as long as a couple has kept building on their relationship during their child-rearing years.

Sex doesn't have to continue, but it doesn't have to end. Assuming that you and your partner want to continue having sex—sildenafil has helped large numbers of older men, and now a growing number of women—and assuming your relationship is strong, it can be a wonderful time in your sexual life. Partners experiencing waning sexual function might also try what Laura has termed VENIS—very erotic noninsertive sex—a program she developed originally to teach adolescents in New York City schools about safer sex, and that grew to be a general sexual enhancement program for all couples, especially those with physical disabilities. Sex is not just about intercourse. All couples, but especially older couples, can give each other sexual pleasure and orgasms through all sorts of activities that don't require erections, even when their range of motion has decreased. Lesbians will certainly attest to this. Since lesbians do not traditionally engage in penile penetration, they tend to pleasure their partners through more touching and exploration without the ultimate goal of penetration. (See chapter 9 for some VENIS techniques.)

In the same way, widowhood doesn't have to mean celibacy, although it's important for a woman to give herself adequate time to grieve before entering into a new relationship. Even then, the new relationship may feel like a betrayal of the previous partner. An older woman may also have to negotiate issues of safer sex that she didn't worry about before. In addition, many older women may find themselves facing sex with only the second partner in their lives—a very stressful prospect. It is perfectly acceptable for a woman to tell her partner how nervous she is. This may actually set a standard of open and positive communication that will not only make her feel safer, but also set the stage for enhanced sexual communication in general. Again, we recommend VENIS as a good alternative to intercourse, and to making certain that you feel safe and comfortable with your partner.

Older women without partners might try self-stimulation if they haven't before. (See chapter 9.) It's never too late to start. Not only does masturbation make you feel better physically and emotionally, sexual arousal and orgasm helps to reduce vaginal atrophy—the drying and thinning of the vaginal wall, which can cause pain during intercourse and vaginal irritation—by increasing lubrication and getting blood flowing to the pelvic region. Once again, the "use it or lose it" adage proves to be true.

Some older women with heart disease worry that the physical stress of sex will put them at risk for heart attacks or strokes. Generally, anyone in good enough condition to walk up two flights of stairs without breathing difficulties and heart pain should be able to have sex. As always, a woman (and her partner) should check with a doctor first. Without complications, a woman should be able to have pleasurable sex, if she wishes, until her last breath.

The Partner

Debra, a 31-year-old mother, and her husband, Scott, had four children, ages 8 to 1, and one of the most common problems of the couples we treat: unequal libido. While Debra was usually too exhausted to think about much less initiate sex, Scott was thinking about it and wanting it all the time. "He could do it twice a day," Debra said.

Busy raising four young children in New York City, Debra was not overly concerned at first about the steady decline in her libido. But her libido had, in fact, been waning for more than six years, ever since the birth of her second child. Debra lost even more interest with the arrival of babies three and four. By the time she came to see us, she was concerned. Her children were now older and required less of her undivided attention, which probably made her notice the problem more. She was overweight from her pregnancies, she said, felt ashamed about her body, and often made excuses to avoid sexual intimacy with her husband. "Or I would pretend I was asleep when he came in," she said. Debra clearly was not interested in sex. Her feelings are not uncommon for women with loss of libido. Some will find themselves working late or busying themselves with night-owl household tasks to avoid any possibility for sexual contact.

Debra's lovemaking with her husband had dropped from four or five nights a week to one or two, hardly a bad average for a couple with a house full of young children, but not at all what her husband wanted. Debra tried consoling herself that things would eventually improve: "I had heard that after having children, your sex drive goes down. I just chalked it up to stress. I figured maybe after the kids were grown and gone, it would get better again. I just didn't put too much priority in it."

Debra's loss of libido was highly frustrating for Scott. At 35, he was not ready to give up his sex life with the hope that it might improve in a decade. He felt unwanted, rejected, and angry. "It was excuse after excuse," he said. At times he worried that there was something physically wrong with Debra and urged her to speak to her gynecologist. Debra refused, saying she was too embarrassed. Other times Scott wondered if his wife might be having an affair. "It's probably the first thing that comes into a guy's head," he said. "But she told me it wasn't me, it was her."

When Debra and Scott came to see us, they were at a stalemate. Still, it was a good sign that they had come in together—many couples don't. Like most couples, they admitted they were nervous at first and said they had never discussed the sexual problems in their marriage with anyone but each other. "It's one of those things that guys don't usually talk to other guys about," Scott said.

Debra and Scott first spoke to Laura, then Debra moved on to our medical evaluation and physiological testing. (See chapter 1.) Debra had never self-stimulated before and was initially embarrassed by the thought of using the vibrator. She felt more comfortable having Scott hold it for her. She had a good sexual response, as shown by her excellent pelvic blood flow, genital engorgement, and vaginal lubrication. She said that she was easily aroused and actually had an orgasm. Since she complained of a dramatic loss of libido, we had suspected that her testosterone levels might be low, but surprisingly her blood tests showed that she was in the normal range. In short, there appeared to be no serious hormonal reason for her loss of libido.

The tests relieved Debra of any fears that there might be something physically wrong with her, but they did raise a whole new set of worries about the source of her problems. "Why can't I get motivated?" she asked.

Underneath all the tension, Debra and Scott seemed to have a loving, committed relationship, with a clear connection to each other. To enhance the foundation of their relationship, we recommended something that should be obvious but that too many couples ignore: the importance of carving out one-on-one quality time. This might consist, for example, of one night a week alone, away from the children. Debra and Scott were in need of adult quality time. Debra especially said she had a hard time turning off the stress of the day.

We referred them to a therapist in the New York area. To temporarily boost arousal, genital sensation, and libido until the root of the problem was identified, we also prescribed a low-dose testosterone cream and sildenafil. We hoped that Debra could use the medications on a short-term basis until the relationship stabilized.

Simultaneously, Debra and Scott started working on their relationship. They both said they were pleased that they at last had their sexual problems out in the open. "It was a relief in a way," Debra said. "As long as we keep talking, it feels good." Debra and Scott are now trying to make more time for each other, although it's difficult when they don't get their children to bed until nine or ten. But recently they told us they found a baby-sitter and spent an entire Thursday together. Scott also says he's more willing to talk about sex. "It has made me a little more open toward the topic," he said, "although I'm not going to say the floodgates are open and that I can talk about it with anybody." Debra and Scott are still working on their relationship, but feel very good about the progress they've made. "It's definitely much better," Debra said. This is a good example of the combination of therapy, counseling, and medical intervention, which had a positive impact on the couple.

Treating a Relationship

Sexuality at its core is a couples issue. Although the purpose of our book is to help the woman, the reality is that relationships are composed of two people and that if one is having sexual problems the other probably is, too. This includes homosexual partners; couple problems are not unique to heterosexuals.

In this chapter we focus on the partner. We'll explore how a woman's sexual problems can adversely affect her partner, and what can be done. We'll also briefly explore problems unique to men, and what their women partners can do to help. It's important to emphasize, though, that in treatment we don't focus on "his" problem or "her" problem. We now know it's "their" problem. Our goal is to treat a relationship.

Getting help early is essential. Since sex is central to intimacy, when a couple is not having sex, or finds it frustrating or difficult, a rift can rapidly develop in the relationship. It's common, and completely normal, for a partner to withdraw or angrily act out. Men especially seem to take a partner's lack of interest or enjoyment as a personal rejection. This is in part why we believe that many women feel compelled to fake orgasms and pretend to be aroused. They are afraid to let their partners down. (Love scenes in the movies that show women loudly in the throes of ecstasy every time they have sex are not accurate representations of reality.) Other women cope with desire problems by avoiding sexual opportunities, anything to avoid having to say no. Most do say yes to sex from time to time, but only because they feel so bad for their partners.

Ideally, a couple should seek treatment together. The good news is that many do. In our practice, Laura usually begins first with the woman, alone. She takes a sexual history, asks about the nature of the problem and how it is affecting her relationship and her life. Then the partner joins in. Laura asks for his or her description of the problem and how he or she perceives it as affecting the relationship. From these conversations, Laura gets an initial sense of how a couple interacts. Sometimes, as with Debra and Scott, we feel it is appropriate for the woman to undergo our physiological testing, but not always. It depends on what the complaints are, what the woman wants, and how much the problem appears to be based on emotional and relationship issues. But even if we suspect that it's largely psychological, some women like Debra insist on the medical testing to assure themselves that there is nothing physiologically wrong.

Our goal is to identify the root of the problem. We need to know if a woman's lack of libido is due to a physical problem, or stress, conflict, or feelings of vulnerability. Or is it simply the result of a woman not getting the sexual stimulation she needs from her partner? All female sexual function complaints can have physiological or psychological causes or both, and all are complicated by the dynamics of the relationship.

To answer these questions, we begin by deconstructing the sexual relationship, usually with a combination of couples and sex therapy. Couples therapy is a form of talk therapy, with the goal of resolving conflict in a relationship. Sex therapy is also talk therapy, but is directed at solving sexual difficulties or sometimes a very specific sexual problem—for example, a lack of libido, a lack of arousal, or early ejaculation.

In sex therapy, Laura asks the couple to refrain from intercourse for a period of time during the initial course of treatment, but gives them "homework" assignments each week, with the goal of rebuilding the sexual relationship from scratch. As we explained in chapter 6, she asks the couple to start out at home with sensual touching, and then slowly build up over the weeks to more intimate and intense sexual contact. Each completed "homework" session is discussed with Laura before another one is assigned. A typical homework assignment may include asking one partner to touch the other without the goal of orgasm. Laura in fact used that assignment for Jill and Mike, the couple mentioned in chapter 6 who had problems with Jill's lack of libido and anxiety during sex. Under instructions from Laura, Jill was able to tell Mike if she was becoming anxious during arousal. That way Mike could ease off the stimulation and make Jill feel more in control. With improved communication and repeated sessions, the goal was for Jill to eventually get through the exercise without anxiety and move on to another level of intimacy. The exercise also helped Jill and Mike diagnose where specific problems may have started in their sexual relationship.

In fact, that's exactly what happened. As their sex therapy progressed, and as Jill's anxiety lessened, it started to become evident to both that the problems were not only about Jill. Mike had fears of rejection and could get extremely anxious himself when initiating sexual activity. As a result, he could be too sexually brusque and assertive with Jill, which in turn made her anxious about being inadequate and made her feel out of control. Fortunately, the two were able to recognize and understand the cycle. In Jill's mind, she was no longer the one "at fault." The problem was not hers but theirs.

Laura usually recommends that a couple commit to at least five one-hour sessions, and then reevaluate. Depending on the couple, the therapy can take as long as several years or as little as two to three months. (For more details about couples and sex therapy, see chapter 5.)

One frequent problem we see among heterosexual partners is anorgasmia in the woman coupled with early ejaculation in the man. In other words, the woman is unable to reach orgasm, or has difficulty reaching orgasm, perhaps as a result of the man's early ejaculation. Or perhaps the man wasn't an early ejaculator at first, but has become frustrated or angry that his partner can't reach orgasm, and has become an early ejaculator or experiences erectile dysfunction as a result. The man may internalize his anger, then begin to feel anxious and inadequate himself. That anxiety, commonly called "performance anxiety," although it's more complicated than that, can adversely affect his ability to maintain or achieve an erection. Some men may get a

"What's the point?" attitude and ejaculate early because they feel that it makes no difference if their partners aren't going to have orgasms anyway. It's always a vicious cycle.

One couple we treated recently had problems like this. More than a decade before, Sarah had experienced a very traumatic childbirth, with lacerations and ripping in the vaginal canal, which created extensive scarring and a lack of sensation. Since then, she had found it difficult to become aroused and reach orgasm with intercourse. Before the delivery she had been fine.

Sarah had lost all interest in sex, but she was willing to be sexual for the sake of intimacy, which she still enjoyed. Her husband, Benjamin, however, had a hard time not taking it personally that she couldn't have an orgasm, and began to fixate on the problem, bringing it up in and out of the bedroom. But all the time and effort he was spending on her arousal only made her more anxious and less likely to become aroused at all. He started to feel inadequate as a result and began to find it difficult to maintain his erection. They had gone on in this way for years, and now were close to a separation.

During her physiologic evaluation, Jennifer noted that Sarah actually had low testosterone levels and that her clitoral and vaginal sensation was low, which is also related to decreased testosterone (and estrogen) levels. We began treating her medically with oral methyltestosterone and, with the help of therapy, we hope the cycle can be broken for them.

Sometimes problems don't arise until many years into the relationship. Aging seems to decrease women's sexual desire more than it does that of men, but this is not a hard and fast rule. There can also be long-standing emotional problems with a mature relationship, beyond any physical problems. We frequently see retired couples with newfound time on their hands, for example, who suddenly find themselves facing sexual issues for the first time.

Ann and Charles, a couple in their seventies, came in seeking therapy at the husband's insistence. Charles had always been physically active and had had a number of infidelities over the years. Ann had responded by creating her own world of friends and social connections and separating her life from his. But now her husband's medical problems had curtailed his sports and social activities and made it impossible for him to drive. Suddenly dependent, Charles wanted to rebuild an intimate relationship with his wife. He was still able to have sex. And, he said, he was lonely.

Ann told Laura she wasn't at all sure that she wanted to reconnect with her husband. After nearly a half century of living a parallel life, she was satisfied. She was active in the community, had many friends, and said she had no interest in sex, either with Charles or anyone else. In part, that was because she was postmenopausal and wasn't on hormone replacement therapy. But her reluctance to engage intimately with her husband was also because of the anger she still felt toward him for cutting her off from his life and for all those years of infidelities. She had no interest in making herself emotionally vulnerable to him. She wasn't interested, she said, in taking the risk.

Charles had told Ann that he was so frustrated by her attitude that he was thinking of finding another sexual partner to meet his needs. Ann's complacency was such that she told

Laura she was considering letting him go ahead with his plans. She said she had no desire to be evaluated physically, either in terms of hormone levels or blood flow, nor was she interested in possibly boosting her sexual interest by taking testosterone. Her only concern was the potential complication: What if her husband fell in love, she asked, and wanted to divorce her? She didn't want to live alone, and she didn't want to give up the roommate-companionship part of the marriage.

The couple clearly had to make a decision. Did they want to salvage their relationship and begin a new courtship, or was the relationship too far gone? Laura laid out to them what would be involved emotionally and logistically if they went through couples therapy together. She told them that if they were committed to trying to stay together, they would need to be willing to come in for regular sessions, go back to the source of the anger, and get themselves to the point where they were able to let it go. She said she would do whatever she could to help them save the marriage, but that they had to decide first if they wanted to and were willing to do the necessary work. At this writing, Ann and Charles remain in limbo, unsure of what to do. But Laura continues to meet with them, and their therapy is focused on trying to clarify their goals as individuals and as a couple.

We had a clearer outcome with Ellen, a professional woman in her late fifties. She, too, came to see us because of a husband unhappy over her loss of libido. The couple had been married for more than three decades, lived in the Northeast, had grown children, and theoretically should have been enjoying the increased freedom in their lives. And to a large extent they were: they spent many active weekends skiing, biking, traveling, and visiting friends. "The kids are out of the house, you see yourself getting older, and you think, 'Oh my God, there are all these things I want to do,'" Ellen said. "It's a wonderful time."

Both were caught up in rewarding and demanding full-time jobs and were also spending more time taking care of their home. Ellen readily described herself as a perfectionist. "I don't sit down, ever," she said. There were times when she wondered if her lack of interest in sex was simply because of all the other activities in her life and because, as she put it, "I don't give myself a chance." At night, she said, "I literally collapse into bed." Even vacations, like a recent hiking trip to Italy, were so active that sex was forgotten, at least by her. "You think you're relaxed and you want to have sex," she said, "but you're exhausted."

Although Ellen said she had never considered herself a person with an enormous sex drive—"I was just never one of those women waiting for my husband in a negligee"—she said she had had a satisfying sexual relationship with her husband for most of their marriage. But as she reached menopause in her mid-fifties, she began to notice a gradual waning of interest. Over the past year, she said, it had become especially pronounced. Sex, she said, "is fine, it's nice, it's a nice thing to do. And once I get going, I'm definitely orgasmic." But she just wasn't interested, beyond the need for intimacy and warmth.

Her husband, however, had a strong sex drive and was as interested as he had always been. "He considers himself a very passionate person, and he would like me to share it," Ellen said. Although the two were still having sex on average twice a week, a rate many other couples young or old would welcome, Ellen said she was only participating because her husband wanted it and she needed to feel close to him. "I always tell him, 'Stop worrying about whether I'm as into it as much as you are,'" she said. She also told him to stop worrying about whether or not she had an orgasm. "If I want to, I will," she said. There were also times when she greeted his advances with, "Be my guest, but don't expect me to participate."

Ellen's husband was increasingly unhappy about her lack of interest. Although Ellen stressed that they were able to talk openly about their problems, he didn't come in with her, and it was clear from her descriptions that the two were experiencing tension and stress. But she was reluctant to discuss any conflict with her husband. She also seemed to be having trouble sorting out how much her lack of interest was from her busy schedule and how much was from any resentment she felt toward him for putting sexual pressure on her.

Ellen's blood test results showed that her testosterone levels were low, as we had expected, but Ellen was reluctant to take any form of testosterone supplement because she was nervous about the side effects. She was, however, interested in the possibility of therapy.

Problems Unique to Men

Although we don't typically treat men medically for erectile dysfunction and early ejaculation—we refer them to a colleague such as Dr. Irwin Goldstein, or if they live outside the Boston area to someone elsewhere—we do help the female partners of men who suffer from the conditions. Many women wrongly blame themselves for the problem, thinking that the man is not attracted to her, or that she has done something to offend him, or that she intimidates him. Many more women have no idea about available treatment. Here, then, are descriptions of the two conditions, and what can be done to help.

Erectile Dysfunction or Impotence

Erectile dysfunction is the inability to have or maintain an erection firm enough for intercourse. It has nothing to do with a man's reproductive function. Impotent men can still have orgasms, ejaculate, and produce sperm. It's also important to remember that a man is not considered impotent if he fails on occasion to get an erection, a universal occurrence among all men. But if the problem becomes persistent and begins to cause stress in a relationship, it's probably time to see a doctor for male sexual dysfunction.

Viagra, the brand name of the drug sildenafil, has actually had a double-edged effect on many couples. For many, the male partner's ability to have an erection is a wonderful relief that brings them closer together. For others, certain conflicts seem to emerge.

For instance, some couples who initially struggled with the male partner's erectile dysfunction and went to sex or couples therapy for help were taught to focus on redefining their sexual life without intercourse. As the couples started to learn about and practice these VENIS (very erotic noninsertive sex) behaviors (see chapter 9), they found that their sexual communication and intimacy actually improved. They had to talk more, share more, and take their time with each other. As a result, the female partners of these men actually responded sexually more effectively and were more satisfied, since most women have difficulty reaching orgasm from intercourse alone. These couples were enjoying a full sexual life without intercourse.

When Viagra came into the picture and produced erections in the male partners, things rapidly shifted. Intercourse became the focus again and sex became more goal-oriented. Also, because most men are not effectively educated about how to use Viagra, many do not have confidence that if the Viagra worked, their erectile ability would maintain itself throughout a sexual encounter. In other words, they didn't know that they could focus on their partner's arousal, lose their erection a little bit in the process, and then regain it. Instead, the focus was on the erection and maintaining it, often to the exclusion of the partner's arousal and satisfaction. So for some couples, regaining erectile potential could negatively affect sexuality.

We've also seen couples who had stopped sexual activity when the male lost his erectile function. They withdrew from sex and often from intimacy in general. Now these men try Viagra, find they can achieve an erection, and want to have sex with their partners. However, the female partners have lost the sense of connection and intimacy that they feel is necessary for their interest. Furthermore, menopause or medical variables may have changed a woman's sexual response. So although Viagra may have tremendous benefits, it is crucial that couples are supported throughout the process of starting to have intercourse, or any sexual activity, again.

The causes of impotence are complex, just as they are in women who have difficulty becoming aroused and reaching orgasm. A generation ago, most impotence was thought to be caused by psychological factors. We now know that 90 percent of impotence has physiological roots, whether from heart disease, hypertension, high cholesterol, diabetes, vascular injuries, surgical procedures, smoking, certain medications, or the overuse of alcohol. Aging is probably the biggest factor. By the age of 65, about a quarter of all men have erectile dysfunction.

Prostate cancer surgery is also a major cause of erectile dysfunction, although rates of impotence vary widely depending on the age of the patient, the location of the cancer, the skill of the doctor, and the patient's sexual function before the operation. Some highly skilled doctors who are adept at the "nerve-sparing" surgery claim that 90 percent of their patients under the age of 65 recover erectile function within a year and a half after the operation. But nationally, among all ages, a study by the Fred Hutchinson Cancer Research Center in Seattle found that almost 60 percent of patients were impotent after prostate surgery. Radiation therapy, even in the form of small "seeds" inserted into the prostate, can also lead to impotence, although this method may more typically cause a man to slowly lose erectile function over the course of treatment.

As an oral pill, sildenafil is the easiest and most recognized new treatment for impotence. It works by increasing blood flow to the penis. If sildenafil isn't effective as a first-line therapy, there are other potentially effective but far more invasive treatments, including penile injections and penile implants. Men should discuss these treatments with a urologist or internist. We encourage women to go to the doctor with their partners, and to be active participants in deciding the best course of treatment.

If a man had a "nerve-sparing" operation—that is, if the nerves vital to erection were preserved during the prostate surgery—he may gradually recover erectile function in the months following prostate surgery. Women should be aware that the erection a man has in the first few months after surgery will probably not be as firm as an erection he may achieve later. A man will also need more direct stimulation of the penis to achieve an erection than he did before. Some urologists are giving sildenafil to the patients immediately following prostate surgery to increase blood flow to the penis (at night during REM sleep, since they are not having intercourse right after surgery). The theory is that increasing penile blood flow helps prevent damage to the nerves and vascular tissue.

Dr. Patrick C. Walsh, Professor and Chairman of the Brady Urologic Institute at Johns Hopkins University, is the creator of nerve-sparing prostate surgery for men. In his patient-oriented book, *The Prostate: A Guide for Men and the Women Who Love Them,* he recommends that men use whatever erection they have to attempt vaginal penetration because vaginal is the best form of stimulation. Once men achieve penetration, they'll often notice that their erections get harder. Dr. Walsh also recommends that men at first attempt intercourse standing up, which can lead to firmer erections. (After prostate surgery blood may still flow into the penis, but the veins may leak and be unable to trap blood inside. Standing up helps solve this "venous leak" problem because the blood has to travel all the way back to the heart, which takes longer than if a man is lying down.

Even if a man is unable to have an erection, from prostate surgery or other problems, sex and couples therapy can help. Laura works first to address what is essentially grief over the loss of intercourse as a part of a couple's intimate life. As is the case with any major loss, it's important for couples to work through the common stages of denial, anger, and acceptance. A man often sees his impotence as a kind of death, as a central part of him that's gone. He may become depressed and withdraw, from both sex and the relationship itself.

Reaching the acceptance stage for impotence of course doesn't take as long as for the death of a loved one. But just as with death, it's in the acceptance stage that couples are able to incorporate the change into their lives. At this point a couple can build on other components of their sexuality beyond intercourse. Laura encourages them to try different sexual activities—manual stimulation, mutual masturbation, oral-genital stimulation, genital kissing, the use of a vibrator. Again, impotence simply means that a man can't get an erection firm enough for vaginal penetration. He may still achieve orgasms as before, although if he's had prostate surgery he will often have a "dry ejaculation" without ejaculate fluid because ejaculation occurs backward into the bladder. Laura's goal is to teach couples that what's commonly considered foreplay can also be a "home run," and that sex is a lot more than just intercourse.

Early Ejaculation

Early ejaculation, or premature ejaculation, is a common problem that is far more difficult to define than impotence since it means different things to different couples. Older definitions actually put time limits on it, like less than two minutes after beginning intercourse, or before a specified minimum number of penile thrusts. Another view is that since most women take longer to reach orgasm than men, the majority of men are therefore "early." In our view, ejaculation is considered early when it occurs before intercourse (if that is the goal), or almost immediately or "too soon" after intercourse begins. The interpretation of "too soon" is best determined by the couples themselves.

The two long-standing sex therapy treatments for early ejaculation are the "squeeze" technique and the "stop and start" method. In the squeeze technique, the man or his partner squeezes the tip of the erect penis just below the "head," or coronal ridge, right before ejaculation. "Stop and start" is just as it sounds: during sexual stimulation or intercourse, when a man feels he is close to ejaculating, he stops and withdraws from the woman's vagina. When he feels he has regained control, he begins again. (See chapter 9.)

We have had mixed success, at best, with these two techniques. Jennifer now also prescribes Zoloft, Prozac, or Anafranil, as do many other urologists, when instruction and therapy fail. Although the drugs are normally used to treat depression, sexual dysfunction is actually among their negative side effects, as discussed in chapter 4. That is, the drugs make it difficult for either women or men to reach orgasm. Zoloft and Prozac are serotonin reuptake inhibitors and work by increasing the amount of the chemical serotonin in the brain. Serotonin brightens moods and lessens anxiety, but it also inhibits sexual arousal and ejaculatory response. Anafranil, a tricyclic antidepressant, causes sexual dysfunction in half the patients who take it. The exact mechanism by which it causes dysfunction is unclear.

In early ejaculators, we've found that Zoloft is highly effective in prolonging the stimulation phase without decreasing the sensation of stimulation or the intensity of orgasm. We give it in a low dose—25 milligrams compared to the standard 50 or 100 milligrams used to treat depression. If a man isn't depressed and takes it, it most likely won't have any other effect on him.

One drug that early ejaculators should definitely not take is Viagra. By increasing blood flow and sensation, Viagra will make early ejaculation even earlier.

We also want to address the problem of low libido in men. Our colleague, Dr. Abe Morgantaler, the director of Men's Health in Boston and a urologist who treats low desire in men, says that low sexual desire in men can be a difficult sexual problem to deal with, for both the man and his partner. This is especially true when the low desire represents a change for the man, or if there is a discrepancy between the man and his partner in their levels of desire.

Men may feel intimidated if their partner appears to have a stronger sex drive than they do and inadequate that they are unable to satisfy their lover's sexual needs. Some men think they must perform sexually even when they do not have the desire, which causes resentment and takes away from the pleasurable anticipation that usually accompanies sex. Ultimately, if a man worries that his sexuality is lacking, he can become quite despondent and think that he is "less than a man."

A woman may be hurt because she feels that she is no longer considered attractive or sexy by her partner. Sometimes a woman will worry that her man has found an outside lover because of his diminished interest in her. But even if the woman feels secure in her partner's desire for her, the lack of sexual interest can cause problems.

There are three main causes of low desire in men:

psychological problems, such as depression, stress, or interpersonal conflicts within the relationship; medication side effects; and hormone deficiency.

Male mice that have been stressed by electric shocks will show no interest in sex when caged with a female, whereas male mice that have not been stressed will actively attempt to mate with the female. Sometimes the first sign of depression in men is that they lose their interest in activities that previously gave them pleasure, such as sex. If there have been struggles in the relationship, particularly about such sexual issues as impotence, a man's brain shuts off its sexual juices, almost as a protective mechanism to avoid further embarrassment.

Many medications can cause diminished desire. Prominent among these are the antidepressants and some high blood pressure medications, such as beta-blockers.

One of the more treatable causes of low desire in men is low levels of testosterone. Testosterone acts on the sexual center in the brain to "turn on" the body for sex. Testosterone levels commonly decline in men as they age. Erections and ejaculation may be normal, but some men may notice that they think about sex less, and that it takes longer for them to "recharge" after having sex.

Treatment depends on the cause of the problem and on the relationship. Counseling or psychotherapy are effective treatments for depression or relationship issues. Stress reduction may be effective in some situations. If no medical cause is present, it is critical that the partner comes to accept and respect the man for who he is and what he offers the relationship so that he feels valued and loved. At the same time, the couple should find ways to maximize their shared sexual pleasure. Weekends and vacations, when stress is reduced, are good times to resharpen the edge of a sexual relationship.

If medication appears to be the cause of low desire, it is important to speak with the prescribing physician to see if another medication could be substituted. And if there has been a change in the man's libido over time, it is important to check testosterone levels, since testosterone treatment is highly effective if this is the problem.

Same Sex Couples

As we noted earlier in this chapter, the affect of sexual dysfunction on a couple is not unique to heterosexuals. Pam and Susan had been together for five years when they came to see us. Sex had always felt very natural to them and they had engaged in sexual activity on a regular basis. However, when Susan reached menopause and started estrogen replacement, she noticed that while her lubrication was fine, her genital sensation and response were not. As a result, she became less interested in sexual activity. Susan didn't seem to be facing any significant emotional struggles in her life.

Pam was not sure what to make of Susan's lack of interest. Although she missed their sexual contact, she did not try to initiate sexual activity.

Laura met with the couple and found that they did communicate well overall, but not as well about sex. Pam was really struggling with how to handle Susan's loss of interest. She not only personalized it, worrying that Susan was no longer attracted to her, but said she found it very difficult to be assertive in their sex life.

This is a problem we often see in lesbian relationships. Since women are typically conditioned not to be sexually assertive (that's a man's right), when two women are in a relationship the sexual roles can be very confusing, not only in dating but in longer-term relationships as well. Susan and Pam did not really face this issue until Susan's lack of interest tipped the balance of their relationship.

When we tested Susan, we found her testosterone levels to be extremely low. Jennifer prescribed testosterone replacement therapy. Laura worked with the couple on their sexual communication skills, regarding this issue and their sex life in general. Once Susan's testosterone was replaced, the couple's sexual relationship improved tremendously.

Problems You Can Work On Yourselves

It's not uncommon for couples of any age to find themselves in a sexual and relationship stalemate. We don't want to suggest that couples or sex therapy is the necessary first stop. It may be more than you need, more expensive than you can afford, or not available in your area. Or it may make you uncomfortable.

So what should you do, for example, if you and your partner are having mediocre or frustrating sex once a month or less, and only for the maintenance of the relationship?

In trying to resolve problems on your own, the first rule is to set aside time to talk about what's bothering you. It seems obvious, but it's amazing how few people really do this. Couples can also try educational videos and books and experiment with what they learn. Always, always communicate with each other along the way. (And please also see chapter 9 for ways to enhance your sexual arousal.)

The most important factor is that both partners agree that they need to work on a problem. If your partner is dismissive at first, keep trying. Some men who act impatient with a partner's problems are really feeling insecure and taking it personally that their partners are not responding sexually. They simply don't want to consider that they may have a role in the problem.

If your partner remains uninterested in helping you with your sexual problems, we don't want to say that you should find another partner. But in this case, we do strongly suggest that you seek help for what probably are a host of other problems in the relationship.

Finally, since there may be medical and physiologic reasons for your or your partner's sexual function problems, we highly recommend that you discuss your symptoms with a physician. If he or she is unable to address the problem, you should ask to be referred to someone who is, and do not take no for an answer. Don't forget, sexuality is an integral component of general wellness and health, and you deserve sexual satisfaction and intimacy.

CHAPTER EIGHT

Exercise, Sex, and Longevity

Exercise is important to a person's sexual health. Sex, in turn, is important to a person's overall health and perhaps even to a person's longevity, potentially adding years to one's life span. In other words, exercise is good for sex and sex is good for you. The two subjects are clearly related and we'll explore both here.

Fortunately, a significant amount of research has been done on the benefits of exercise for a woman's general health and wellness, especially cardiac health. Unfortunately, very little of it has focused on the role exercise plays in enhancing or maintaining a woman's sexual health. The effects of sex on female longevity are also poorly understood. As with so much else in our field, we expect that to change soon. In the meantime, here is what we know now.

The Role of Exercise in Sexual Health

In late 1998 Carla Dionne, a mother of three in her early forties who had always enjoyed a satisfying sex life, underwent uterine artery embolization, a relatively new procedure for the treatment of fibroids. In Carla's case, the procedure was successful and the fibroids, noncancerous growths on or near the uterus that can cause pain and bleeding, disappeared. (See chapter 4 for more information on fibroids.) But the aftereffects Carla experienced in terms of her sexual response were completely unexpected. She was shocked when she found, during her first sexual encounter following the procedure, that she had almost no sensation in her pelvic area during sex. Carla had previously experienced great satisfaction during intercourse from deep penetration. She also experienced strong uterine and pelvic floor contractions during orgasm. Following the procedure, she found it more difficult to have an orgasm, and when she could have one, she described them as shorter in duration and less intense, nothing like she had experienced before.

As part of her investigation into what might be the cause for sexual difficulties, Carla contacted us. Based on her symptoms and the sudden change in her sexual response, we suspected that the embolization may have affected the branches of her uterine or vaginal arteries and the blood flow to her pelvic region. As we discussed in chapter 4, during an embolization, small particles of plastic, called polyvinyl alcohol or PVA, are injected into the uterine artery. This blocks the blood supply feeding the fibroids. Some women, like Carla, who experience pelvic floor orgasms before the procedure, report a loss of uterine contractions and sensation after this procedure.

In an attempt to get some of her strength back, and also to improve her mood, Carla started going to the gym. For five evenings a week, she did aerobic exercises and lifted weights. Then she finished off each exercise session with 15 minutes of sit-ups and pelvic lifts.

Carla had always known that exercise was important to her health and well-being, and so she wasn't surprised when both her strength and mood improved. But something else happened, too. After two hours at the gym in the evening, she found her sexual energy and response greatly improved. The warmth of her body and the sensation of blood pumping through her arteries made her full of desire, a feeling that lasted several hours after she returned home, and made it easier for her to become aroused and reach orgasm.

"If I haven't worked out, it's just a lengthier process for me to get there in terms of blood flow and lubrication," she said. "When I come home, I'm warm. The muscles have been stretched, the blood flow is there. It facilitates sex and it just makes it a whole lot easier. Faster, too."

Carla is now the executive director of the National Uterine Fibroid Foundation, and she has asked us to be members of her advisory board. (For more information on her work and her Web site, see the Resources section in chapter 9.) Carla frequently tells women who have had sexual response problems after embolizations and other pelvic surgery that exercise is extremely helpful, assuming, that is, that the women are healthy and that exercise does not cause pain. Limited aerobic activity is enough; you don't need to go for heavy duty workouts at the gym. Do whatever makes you feel good—swimming, cycling, brisk walking, whatever works for you.

The role of exercise in improving physical and emotional health is by now well known, but the long list of its benefits bears repeating: regular exercise plays a major role in preventing heart disease, high blood pressure, strokes, diabetes, and osteoporosis. Exercise may also help to prevent colon, endometrial, and breast cancer. Exercise reduces stress and anxiety, can help reduce depression, helps to maintain normal weight, builds muscle strength, and helps improve a woman's body image. It lowers the "bad" cholesterol in your blood, the harmful low-density lipoprotein, or LDL, that causes the buildup of fat deposits in the arteries. Exercise also raises the levels of "good" cholesterol, the high-density lipoprotein, or HDL, which prevents fat buildup in the arteries.

We are learning more each day about how important exercise is to sexual function. It helps in two important ways. First, exercise contributes to relaxation and a sense of well-being—both crucial to getting in the mood for sex—with the release of endorphins, the "feel good" chemicals. During exercise, the body produces endorphins, which act on the brain to block pain and create feelings of exhilaration. That is why many people often feel happier and calmer after a session of exercise.

Second, exercise—particularly vigorous aerobic exercise—increases blood flow throughout the body including to the pelvic area and genitals, where it can act as a kind of "natural" Viagra. As is the case with Viagra, increased blood flow to the pelvic region and genitals can improve sensation, lubrication, arousal, and the intensity of orgasm.

Dr. Irwin Goldstein and his colleagues recently published the findings of a nine-year study following nearly 600 men with erectile dysfunction problems. They found that men who were already active and those who started exercising during the study were at a lower risk for incidents of erectile dysfunction. Dr. Goldstein believes that one of the most important implications of the study is that men can reduce their risk for dysfunction even if they wait until middle age to become physically active.

To understand why, it's important to know what happens physiologically during vigorous exercise for 20 minutes or more. In essence, the heart, the body's most important muscle, gets a workout by more forcefully pumping blood and making it circulate faster throughout the body. At the same time, the work of the heart delivers oxygen and nutrients to all parts of the body and takes away wastes more quickly. Over time, sustained, aerobic exercise (like jogging, swimming, skiing, biking, or fast walking) makes the walls of the heart grow thicker and stronger, allowing it to pump more blood with less effort. Regular aerobic exercise also increases the number and size of blood vessels in the tissues and so increases the blood supply to all parts of the body.

We are in no way recommending that a woman with sexual dysfunction immediately go out and sprint a mile before having sex. As always, a woman—particularly a sedentary one—should check with her doctor before embarking on any exercise program.

In fact, we ourselves have never prescribed exercise per se as the sole treatment for sexual dysfunction, although we strongly believe that regular exercise is an important part of a woman's overall sexual health. Over the years we have seen many times that exercise helps a flagging sex life in individuals without other adverse factors to explain their problems. Laura has had patients, for example, who actually experienced orgasms during the jumping, stretching, or leg-lifting portions of aerobics classes. Orgasms can occur during these situations because the women's genitals are directly stimulated by leg positions during exercise. The increased blood flow to the area, combined with the clenching of the pelvic floor muscles, contributes to the heightened sensations.

We've also treated patients who, like Carla, had diminished

sexual response but who saw significant improvement in sensation and arousal after exercising. (This is true in men as well, who sometimes report a greater ability to achieve erections after exercise.) One of our patients, a 38-year-old dentist, told us that the only way that she could reach orgasm by self-stimulation or with her partner was by doing leg lifts and tightly clenching her buttocks 30 minutes prior to sex. She discovered this, she told us, after an exercise class—when she had her first orgasm.

Research supports the findings that we have seen in our patients. Dr. Cindy M. Meston, assistant professor of clinical psychology at the University of Texas, has done some of the most interesting and persuasive work in the field. Although doctors have long understood the role that exercise plays in creating the good mood conducive to satisfying sex, Dr. Meston chose to look directly at the effects of acute exercise on a woman's physiological sexual response.

In the mid-1990s while she was a graduate student at the University of British Columbia in Vancouver, Canada, Dr. Meston, along with Dr. Boris B. Gorzalka, studied 35 women, ranging in age from 18 to 34, who were all involved in heterosexual relationships and had no history of sexual dysfunction. Dr. Meston found that along with a sexual stimulus—in this case, an erotic video—exercise "facilitates" physiological sexual arousal in women. Specifically, Dr. Meston found that when women watched the erotic video after exercise, as compared to watching it before exercise, their genital engorgement increased 168 percent. Genital engorgement was measured using vaginal photoplethysmography. This technique, like Duplex Doppler ultrasound, measures changes in blood flow to the vagina.

Dr. Meston conducted her study in two parts. In the first

session, each woman went separately into a private room and inserted the photoplethysmograph into her vagina. The photoplethysmograph is a penlight-like device, predating the techniques we now use at our clinic, that measures change in the redness of vaginal tissues and also records the volume of blood flow. With the device inserted, each woman then viewed a neutral three-minute travelogue followed by a three-minute erotic film of a heterosexual couple engaging in foreplay and intercourse. Changes in blood flow and heart rate were monitored and recorded.

In a second session, each woman cycled on a stationary bicycle for 20 minutes. Her heart rate was constantly monitored so that an experimenter could adjust the pressure on the pedals throughout the session to make sure that she was exercising at 70 percent of her maximum heart rate—a vigorous level of activity and one that had to be the same for each woman, regardless of physical condition, to make the study consistent. After that, each woman inserted the photoplethysmograph, then watched the travelogue and erotic video as before. Changes were recorded.

Each woman was also asked to fill out a questionnaire after each session to judge her perception of the level of sexual response. Interestingly, there was no statistical difference in these subjective ratings of sexual response between the exercise and no-exercise sessions. In other words, although dramatic changes in genital blood flow were recorded following exercise, the women did not subjectively notice a difference in their responses. Dr. Meston theorized that the women may not have attributed physiological changes brought on by arousal, such as heavy breathing and a fast heartbeat, because they were already experiencing these symptoms due to the exercise.

Despite the absence of subjective changes in sexual responses due to exercise, the objective increase in genital engorgement, as demonstrated by the photoplethysmography after exercise, was striking. These findings led Dr. Meston to conclude that exercise can physiologically prepare—in essence, activate—your body for sexual activity. Such a conclusion, Dr. Meston adds, causes a predictable reaction when she speaks of it to young men: they invariably say they'll start hanging around the gym on the lookout for willing women. To which Dr. Meston says, "No, they still have to perceive you as an erotic stimulus. And that's the hard part." In other words, although physical activity may prepare the body for sex, you still need, as with Viagra, a psychological cue. Desire still needs to come from the primary sex organ, the brain. One of Dr. Meston's theories is that the reason couples often have intense sex after arguments is because their heart rate, blood pressure, and endorphins are all elevated, a physiological residue of anger, but they are at the same time psychologically in tune because they've made up.

The Role of Sex in Overall Health and Longevity

Just like exercise, sex can reduce stress, enhance mood, and increase self-esteem. In fact, psychiatrists sometimes prescribe both sex and exercise to anxious patients. In addition, regular sex over time supports the concept of "use it or lose it." The more sexually active a woman is, especially into her menopausal years, the better her genital blood flow and vaginal health will remain. Sex helps keep up a regular blood flow through the pelvic arteries, which helps to keep the arteries and genital tissue in shape. In this regard, regular sexual activity during menopause can also help to reduce vaginal atrophy—the drying and thinning of the vaginal wall, which can cause pain during intercourse and vaginal irritation—by increasing blood flow and lubrication.

A number of studies have suggested that people who have sex more often live longer. There are, however, problems with some of the methodology in these studies, particularly because the researchers didn't consider other health factors. As a result, the studies so far show only a correlation between sex and longevity, not a cause-and-effect relationship. Worse, the most recent large study doesn't include women. But the results are still worth considering.

The Duke First Longitudinal Study of Aging, begun at Duke University in the 1950s, looked at 270 men and women over a span of 25 years. The study found that the frequency of intercourse was a significant predictor of longevity for men while enjoyment of intercourse was a predictor for women—indicating, the researchers surmised, that quantity is more important to men and quality is more important to women. In either case, the findings seemed to suggest that having more sex made people live longer, either because of the physical activity, the emotional gratification, or both. But the researchers also pointed out that the findings—at least as they related to men—might simply reflect the fact that healthier men tend to be more sexually active.

A later study in Sweden associated the early cessation of intercourse with an increased mortality risk in men, while another study found sexual dissatisfaction in women to be a risk factor in heart attacks. (In that study, an underlying cause of the women's sexual dissatisfaction was early ejaculation and impotence in their male partners.)

Findings from the more recent Caerphilly study, which followed 2,512 men from the Welsh town of Caerphilly and five adjacent villages, found what the researchers called "an inverse relation between orgasmic frequency and mortality"—even, the researchers said, when the results were adjusted for age, social class, smoking patterns, and overall health. In a 1997 article about the study in the *British Medical Journal*, the researchers—George Davey Smith, Stephen Frankel, and John Yarnell—concluded that men who had orgasms twice a week or more had lower rates of mortality from all causes. They also suggested, with some amusement, that the results of the study might lead to public health campaigns urging citizens to have sex, similar to those that advocate eating five helpings of fruits and vegetables a day. "The disappointing results observed in health promotion programs in other domains," the researchers said, "may not be seen when potentially pleasurable activities are promoted."

We should mention that having orgasms isn't necessary to preserve sexual function. In many eastern traditions, particularly in tantric sex (a form of sexual activity that is based on breathing, eye contact, body centering, and other Eastern philosophies about sex), sexual contact and arousal are considered extremely healthy, but orgasm is not always necessary nor in the best interest of a man's longevity.

Dr. Michael F. Roizen, a gerontologist at the University of Chicago and the author of *Real Age: Are You as Young as You Can Be?* calls the Caerphilly study "the strongest proof we have that sex can actually help us to get younger and stay younger." By his calculations, the study shows that having sex twice a week can add nearly two years to a person's life. Having satisfying sex once a day, Dr. Roizen says, can add eight.

CHAPTER NINE

Helping Yourself

W e've tried to be as helpful as possible in explaining the causes of and treatments for sexual dysfunction and how you can focus on yourself and reclaim your sex life. But many times what is most needed is practical information and basic techniques. We've found that even people who are completely satisfied with their sex lives can use a little creativity. Here, then, are some "how to" hints and techniques for enhancing your arousal and sexual pleasure.

How to Enhance Your Sexual Arousal and Pleasure in General

❖ The first task is to let go of a goal-oriented approach. Try not to focus on orgasm as the end point. Focus instead on sensuality. Specifically, try to enhance awareness of your other erogenous zones—lips, eyelids, inner thighs, buttocks, back, neck, feet, ears—with touching, kissing, erotic touch, and light massage. Often when we let go of orgasm-focused, or intercourse-focused, sex, the act becomes much more a reflection of intimacy, connection, eroticism, and arousal. Sex can be much more fun with much less pressure to perform. If a woman becomes anxious when a sexual experience begins, worrying that she won't be able to reach orgasm, it is likely that her body will respond to her anxiety, her blood vessels will constrict, and her arousal will diminish.

❖ Make sure that you keep the lines of communication with your partner open.

❖ Allow yourself the luxury of fantasies. Don't be ashamed of your fantasies and try to be creative. Some women enjoy using their private fantasies either alone or with a partner. Others like to share them and talk them out. This in part depends on the strength of the relationship and the ease of the communication between partners. Some partners may be threatened by your fantasies about others, while other partners will find fantasies stimulating, too. The thing to remember is that having a fantasy and acting on one are two different things. Most women, as well as men, say that the reason their fantasies are so stimulating is because they are something that would never happen in real life, nor would they want them to. Fantasies don't have to involve another person or more than one partner. Fantasies can simply be about having sex in different locations. Some of the more popular fantasies we hear about involve the beach or an elevator or an airplane.

❖ Use lubricants. In safer sex, lubricants should be water-based, like K-Y Jelly, Astroglide, and Foreplay. Vaseline,

baby oil, and Crisco can break down the latex in condoms. Nonoxynol-9 is a spermicidal lubricant on many
condoms that is widely believed to kill HIV. However, according to a study presented at the 13th annual AIDS
conference, women who consistently used Nonoxynol-9
nearly tripled their risk of infection, so you should discuss
this option with your doctor. In addition to drugstores,
erotica shops also carry a wide range of water-based lubricants. Some are flavored, some are creamy, some
counteract vaginal dryness, and some cause warm, tingling sensations in the genitals.

❖ Try different kinds of sexual toys or foodstuffs. Some
couples like to use whipped cream, chocolate sauce, or
honey. Others like to engage in light bondage play.
Erotica shops often carry fur-lined Velcro handcuffs, silk
eye masks, feathers, and videos as well as an array of kits
for tantric and other alternative sex play.

❖ Try aromatherapy. Erotica shops carry many scents
thought to enhance energy, relaxation, and sensuality.
Even fresh flowers can help set the mood. Some oils also
induce warmth and tingling that may accentuate arousal.

❖ Pay attention to your environment. Many women are
context-oriented and need to feel comfortable and safe
before they can enjoy sex. Take a bubble bath, light candles, put on soft music. Some women like to wear lingerie
to help them get into a sexy mood. Many women need a
transition period to let go of all the stress in their lives before they can relax and turn their attention to their sexuality. A woman needs to see sex as part of taking care of

herself, not just as something she does for her partner or her relationship.

How to Talk to Your Partner about Sex

The first rule is honesty. Let your partner know what you like and want, but never, ever fake an orgasm. It's tempting, it's easy, and lots of women do it, but it gets you into trouble by setting up a negative cycle that may be difficult to get out of. True, your partner wants you to have an orgasm, and a woman often believes that by faking an orgasm she's doing her partner a favor. But the downside is that she's devaluating her own sexuality. You're also depriving yourself and your partner of the opportunity of discovering what pleases you.

When and if a woman who has been faking orgasms does want to try to enhance her sexual response, the act of confessing that she was faking can be devastating to her partner, often adding to the problem and causing harm to the relationship. If you have been faking orgasms, it is never too late to tell your partner, but be prepared for your partner to feel deceived. It may take time to repair your relationship in order to move on to your own sexual healing.

If telling your partner is simply impossible, another option may be to modify your behavior by expressing your need to change your activities to enhance your sexual pleasure. This may work in some cases, but reaching orgasm with a partner requires cooperation and communication. It is a joint effort that both partners should ideally be invested in.

The far better alternative is to tell your partner what to do to sexually satisfy you from the beginning. Only 20 to 30

percent of women have orgasms as a result of vaginal penetration alone; most need direct stimulation of the clitoris for
an orgasm. If you need added stimulation, show your partner what feels good, or learn to feel comfortable doing it
yourself. (For tips on how to have an orgasm during intercourse, see pages 206–11.)

Most men learn how to give sexual pleasure to a woman,
if they do at all, from friends (most of whom are misinformed), pornography (most of which has been geared
toward men's arousal, not women's), or high school sex education (typically anatomy and safer sex, not sexual techniques). Clearly, these are not the best sources. Unless a man
is with a woman who is willing to let him know what to do,
he can be with 100 other women and still not have a clue.
Every woman is different, and it's her responsibility to tell a
partner what she likes. One woman we know was preparing
to consummate her relationship with her boyfriend on a romantic vacation in Bermuda and expected that because he
had been with so many other women he would be a great
lover. They had talked often about their past sexual es-
capades and were both looking forward to sharing a sexual
experience together in this romantic environment. To her
amazement, he had no idea of a woman's basic sexual
anatomy. Rather than faking an orgasm, the next day she
drew him a diagram in the pink sand of one of Bermuda's
beaches, sketching out the vagina and clitoris and showing
him how she liked to be touched. Some couples find it helpful to self-stimulate in front of each other; this can also be a
fun alternative to regular intercourse. (For more information
on how to self-stimulate, see pages 202–4.)

Women who feel awkward or embarrassed bringing up
sex with a partner or who are worried they won't say the

right thing or might offend their partner might try introducing educational and erotic videos and books into a relationship. (For suggestions, see our Resources section at the end of this chapter.) Many women find that if they bring a video home, the couple can watch it together, which more easily starts a conversation about sex and the relationship.

For larger discussions about your sexual needs, the best time to talk is probably not during sex. Since it is such an intimate and vulnerable setting, it is easy for a partner to feel criticized and hurt. A woman can provide positive guidance and encouragement when her partner is doing something right and certainly should let him or her know if they are doing something that is uncomfortable or unpleasurable in as soft a way as possible. If you want to talk about it afterward, or you want to introduce a new sexual idea into the relationship, talking about it when you are not in the midst of the sexual act can help to take the pressure off. It also helps to focus only on the positive, such as "I love it when you————," "I would really love it if you would do more————," or "It would really be exciting to try————."

How to Do Kegel Exercises

Strengthening the pubococcygeous (pc), or pelvic floor, muscles surrounding the opening of the vagina can help you to intensify arousal and orgasm. It will allow you to grasp the penis better, heightening arousal for both you and your partner. Kegel exercises are named for Arnold Kegel, the gynecologist who created them. Doing them every day can strengthen your pelvic floor muscles, which not only helps bladder control but can lead to more intense orgasms and greater sexual pleasure.

To do Kegel exercises, first identify the pelvic floor muscles by clenching as though to stop urination in midstream. These are the muscles you need to exercise. Practice by stopping and then starting the flow when you urinate. When you're not urinating, practice contracting the muscles. You can do this anytime, anywhere—lying down, sitting up, standing, at the office, in the car, in line at the grocery store. No one will be able to see what you are doing.

Start out by contracting your vagina for 2 to 3 seconds, repeating 10 times. Repeat the sets of 10 throughout the day. You should do at least 5 sets, or 50 contractions, a day. As your muscles strengthen, gradually extend the time of each contraction to 8 to 10 seconds. The longer you hold the contraction, the more effective the exercise, and the stronger your muscles will become.

Julie Tupler is an R.N. who created a program for pregnant women called Maternal Fitness, which resulted in a book by the same name (see the Resources section at the end of this chapter). We recommend the book to all women, regardless of their childbearing status, because she focuses on enhancing the strength of the entire pelvic floor and inner abdominal muscles. She concentrates her efforts not only on Kegel exercises but on transverse exercises as well (for example, sitting with your back against the wall and slowly sucking in and holding your stomach muscles in an "elevator" fashion). These exercises greatly improve muscle control, fitness, and even sexual response.

How to Self-Stimulate

Masturbation is a natural and healthy expression of sexuality that helps a woman get to know her own body and to learn what pleases her. About 80 percent of women masturbate at least occasionally. Unfortunately, many women don't understand their basic sexual anatomy. Some don't know what their genitals look like. (For help, see chapter 3 on female anatomy.)

To begin, carve out some time for yourself when you are alone, without children, a partner, or other distractions. Some women use videos or fantasies to add to the erotic landscape. Some women like to take a bath or shower first, or light candles and put on music. Prepare lubricants, which greatly enhance sexual arousal. Some women like to use water-based gels, like K-Y Jelly or more exotic concoctions from erotica shops. (See our Resources section at the end of this chapter.) Others simply moisten their fingers with saliva.

Next, lie down on your back, or lie down on your stomach, or sit up. Just as with sex with a partner, there is no "correct" position. If this is the first time, you might want to look at your genitals first by spreading your legs and using a mirror. A hand-held mirror works well, but any mirror will do. If you are uncomfortable looking at yourself, you may want to start by simply feeling your genitals with your fingers. If that makes you uncomfortable, feel your genitals with your hand. Start by stroking and touching your entire body with your hands, feeling your breasts, stomach, arms, inner thighs, and other erogenous zones. Explore and practice touching your genitals in different areas. Stroke the clitoris, either directly or on the pubic bone right above. Touch the labia majora, the labia minora, the urethra, and the perineum. Get a sense of ownership and agency over your body. The only goal is to get to know your body and what feels good.

Experiment with different kinds of touch—harder, softer, quicker, slower. Every woman is different. Some women like to gently and rhythmically rub the clitoris itself, with one or more fingers, slowly increasing the intensity in a way that feels pleasurable. Others like to rub the larger area around the clitoris, or exert pressure on the pubic bone above it and the urethra below it. This may be combined with or instead of vaginal stimulation, which many women enjoy as well. This can be achieved using a finger or a vibrator and involves penetration and stimulation of the areas around and inside the vagina. A woman can rub up and down, or back and forth, or round and round, experimenting with pressure. Some women also like to stimulate the area in and around their anuses. Practice tightening and loosening your pelvic floor muscles while stimulating yourself. And breathe deeply; this will help to relax and center you, and the air exchange in your body during deep breaths will help to enhance arousal. Again, don't make orgasm the goal, just focus on increasing the stimulation and doing what feels good.

Some women masturbate by crossing their legs and exerting rhythmic pressure on their genital area. Many women like to rock their pelvises while masturbating. Continue to experiment and see what feels good for you. Allow yourself to enjoy the process.

Many women who don't like the idea of touching themselves directly or who prefer more intense stimulation use a vibrator. (However, comfort and ease with your body is an important component of sexual arousal.) A vibrator is helpful because it provides a level of stimulation that no human can produce. Many women (and men) are under the misconception that a vibrator will cause a lack of interest in a partner. It's true that orgasm may happen more easily with a vibrator, but sex is about a lot more than orgasm. No machine can replace intimacy, body contact, and human connection. Ideally, a vibrator can be used to incorporate all a woman learns about her body during self-stimulation into a relationship. There are many different kinds of vibrators. Some directly stimulate the clitoris and can be used during intercourse with a partner. Others are penile shaped for use inside the vagina. Some women like to insert a penile-shaped vibrator while they self-stimulate their clitorises. (For details and availability, see our Resources section at the end of this chapter.)

After you've become comfortable with masturbation, share what you've learned with your partner. If you feel comfortable, let your partner watch you self-stimulate, then teach your partner how to stimulate you in a way you enjoy. Start out by guiding his or her hand, then provide ongoing direction. If you are without a partner, self-stimulation is usually a worthwhile end in itself for maintaining healthy sexuality.

Two excellent references for learning more about self-stimulation are *Becoming Orgasmic* by Julia R. Heiman and Joseph Lopiccolo and *Sex for One* by Betty Dodson, both of which are available in book and video formats. Both provide details about women's bodies and details about how to self-stimulate.

How to Practice Very Erotic Noninsertive Sex (VENIS)

VENIS, or very erotic noninsertive sex, is sex without penetration. It involves broadening your ideas of what sex is beyond intercourse to focus on non–goal-oriented activities. In other words, VENIS aims to turn foreplay into a home run. This may involve a whole range of activities, which may or may not lead to orgasm, but all of which can be experienced as erotic and stimulating: erotic wrestling with maximum body and genital contact, massaging each other with oils or other materials, manual stimulation, light bondage with feathers or fur, mutual masturbation, erotic dancing, intercourse between breasts or buttocks, and body kissing are just some of the possibilities.

Many couples find that engaging in VENIS activities takes the pressure off when they are having difficulty with intercourse due to erectile dysfunction or vaginal dryness. Other couples who enjoy VENIS simply like adding variations on the common theme of intercourse. VENIS is also a great safer sex alternative because the majority of VENIS activities do not involve the exchange of bodily fluids. VENIS requires verbal and body communication between partners, which may feel intimidating at first. However, most couples who have incorporated VENIS into their sexual lives report that their sexual satisfaction and their sexual communication skills have vastly improved as a result.

How to Have an Orgasm during Intercourse

Most women don't have orgasms with intercourse alone, and there is no one orgasm that is better than another. However, for the many women who come to us and say they would like to have an orgasm during intercourse, here are descriptions of positions and techniques that may help a woman have an orgasm with a male partner during coitus:

❖ Try the missionary position with a pelvic tilt: this position helps the penis to hit the site of the G-spot, or what we now know is the part of the clitoris that extends into the anterior, or belly-side, vaginal wall. You should be on your back, beneath the man, with your pelvis tilted upward. Your vulva should be angled so that it presses flat against your partner's pelvic bone and causes friction on the clitoris, urethra, and labia minora. Experiment with different angles, which shift the angle of the penis, to see what works best. It helps to place one or more pillows beneath your buttocks, or to have your partner lift up your buttocks with his hands. See figure 9.1.

❖ Try the coital alignment technique, or CAT, advanced by psychotherapist Edward W. Eichel. Your partner should lie across your body without supporting himself on his elbows, minimizing stress in his upper torso. He should shift his pelvis forward from the standard missionary position to what's called the pelvic-override position, making sure the base of his penis makes direct contact with the clitoris. You and your partner should then engage in a rhythmic, coordinated back and forth rocking motion

Figure 9.1 Missionary position with pelvic tilt

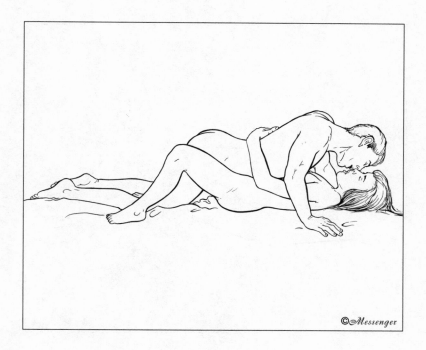

©Messenger

rather than penile thrusting. You should lead the upward motion while your partner leads the downward motion, making sure that the penile-clitoral connection is constantly maintained through pressure and counterpressure. See figure 9.2.

❖ Get on top. This allows a woman to adjust the position of her pelvis and to more fully control the friction of the base of the penis as it rubs against her labia and clitoris. This can lead to a clitoral orgasm. She may also use the position to allow for deep thrusting into her vagina, which can lead to stimulation of the cervix and a pelvic

Figure 9.2 Coital alignment technique (CAT)

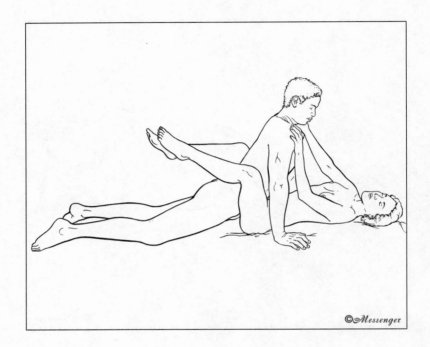

©Messenger

floor orgasm. (See Stimulate the cervix, p. 210.) This position can be carried out with your partner lying down or sitting and can involve a rocking-chair motion that many couples find stimulating due to the deep penetration and clitoral stimulation. See figure 9.3.

❖ Flex your pelvic floor muscles: Kegel exercises, or pulling in on your vagina as if you're trying to stop urination, builds up your pelvic floor, or pc, muscles. (To learn how to do them, see pages 200–201.) Many women flex these muscles during intercourse to get a tighter trip on their partner's penis and to give him greater pleasure. But flexing these muscles, especially if they're well exercised, may give you pleasure as well. The stronger the muscles are, the tighter you'll be able to contract your vagina, which will create greater friction against your partner's penis and more stimulation to the part of your clitoris that lies against the vaginal wall. Try squeezing down throughout intercourse and then especially hard as you feel yourself nearing a climax. Some women report that this gives them an especially intense orgasm. In fact, practicing this exercise through maturity may also diminish the likelihood of urinary leakage later in life.

Figure 9.3   Classic position with woman on top

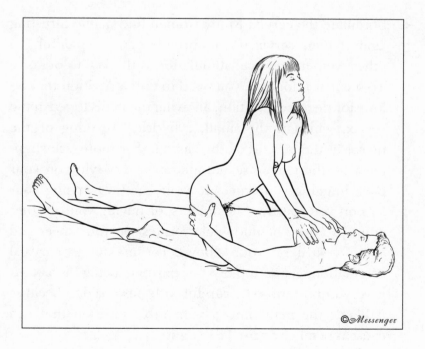

❖ Keep your legs together. In the missionary position, not all pleasurable sex needs to happen while you're spread-eagled. Keeping your legs together can create friction from the penis on the visible clitoral glans and can lead to a clitoral orgasm. Once your partner has inserted his penis into your vagina, squeeze your legs closed and have him place his legs outside yours. He can help by then squeezing your legs further closed with his thighs. It also helps if he can shift his pelvis forward so that he makes his pubic bone cause pressure and friction on your clitoris and labia minora. (See missionary position with pelvic tilt, above.) He should then start thrusting, slowly and evenly, so that his penis rubs the base of the clitoral glans. He can speed up as you become more aroused and near orgasm.

❖ Stimulate the cervix: Many women find penile thrusting against their cervix uncomfortable or even painful. To other women, cervical stimulation is the key to orgasm. To see if it is for you, you need to find a position that allows for deep penetration, allowing the penis to reach the cervix, which is the small, cylindrical opening of the uterus at the far end of the vagina. (For more, see chapter 3 on the female sexual anatomy.) Try lying on your back hugging your knees to your chest, or resting your legs on your partner's shoulders, or having your partner enter you from behind while you rest on your knees and lean forward on your elbows. For maximum cervical stimulation, get on top of your partner, facing his feet. (It is very important to be careful with this position because it bends the penis into a vulnerable position that can cause a penile fracture.) See figure 9.4.

Figure 9.4 Cervical stimulation position

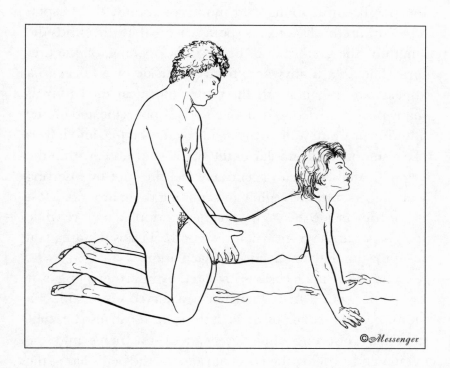

©*Messenger*

How to Ejaculate

There is some controversy over female ejaculation, whether it's possible for a woman to learn how to do it or if it's just a natural ability, and even whether it exists at all. Kim Airs, a sex educator and proprietrix of Grand Opening!, a sexuality boutique in Brookline, Massachusetts, suggests that women can indeed learn how to ejaculate. We'd like to stress, however, that this is just one aspect of sexuality to explore, and not necessary for sexual satisfaction.

Female ejaculation can occur when the internal area

around the urethra is stimulated. The area is also known as the paraurethral sponge or, more commonly, the G-spot. The paraurethral sponge is spongy tissue that surrounds the length of the urethra and the neck, or opening, of the urethra. The area is anywhere from a knuckle of a finger to a knuckle-and-a-half inside the vagina (not near the cervix as many people are led to believe). The G-spot is located on the anterior, or front, wall of the inside of the vagina, and it feels like a smooth spot, similar to the tip of your nose, within the vaginal canal. You can accurately feel the spot by inserting your fingers into the vagina and rotating them around. Most of the area inside the vagina will have a rippled texture while the G-spot at the front will feel smooth. This is the area you want to stimulate to encourage ejaculation.

The area can be easily stimulated by inserting a finger or two (either your own or a partner's), a curved sexual aid, or a vibrator, and pressing up against the spot. It can also be stimulated by inserting only the head of the penis into the vagina and stroking the coronal ridge of the penis along the smooth area. To stimulate this area with your fingers, stroke the area as if you were rubbing the back of the clitoris, making a "come here" motion with your fingers. The motion and slight pressure should make the area swell with fluid, which is gathered in the paraurethral sponge. Physiologically, this is similar to what happens when a penis is stimulated and becomes erect.

Ejaculation can occur when the woman has the sensation that she has an urge to urinate. The sensation is exactly like the feeling of being full. (You may want to eliminate any doubt by urinating before having a sexual encounter, which is a good idea anyway.) If you are hesitant to wet the bed (or wherever else this is happening), you may want to put a few towels underneath you between your hips and your knees.

The next step is to push your pelvic floor muscles outward, as if you were giving birth or pushing out a tampon. This will change the way your vaginal opening looks, and will often display the muscular tissue surrounding the urethra as well. A few drops can dribble out of the vagina, or you may release a large amount of fluid that can come gushing out. The fluid is virtually clear and relatively odorless (although this can change according to a woman's menstrual cycle).

Remember, the quantity of fluid released does not reflect on the pleasure of the sexual experience, nor on any "lack of femininity." Some women ejaculate unintentionally with every sexual encounter, and many women don't ejaculate at all.

How to Perform the Squeeze and Start-and-Stop Techniques for Early Ejaculation

---

Next to erectile dysfunction, early ejaculation may be the most common explanation for failure of a male partner to successfully have intercourse with his partner. Assuming that the man has no medical explanations for his difficulties, there are two basic treatments for early ejaculation in which a man's partner can be involved.

* ❖ In the squeeze technique, a man first starts with self-stimulation, bringing himself almost to the point of

"ejaculatory inevitability." In other words, he uses the squeeze technique right before he feels the need to ejaculate. Most men are able to identify this point. The squeeze technique involves placing the fingers around the head of the penis and putting pressure on the frenulum of the penis—the small, triangular fold of skin on the underside just below the tip, or glans—and just above the coronal ridge, the rim on the front of the penis that separates the glans from the shaft. The squeeze should last about four seconds. When the man feels he is under control, stimulation can continue.

Once a man is able to do this alone, he should do it with his partner present. The next step is intercourse, initially with the woman on top because it puts the man in a better position for the squeeze. The couple should begin with what's called non-demand coitus, or penetration, in which they remain still, without thrusting. If at any time the man feels that he's close to ejaculation, he can quickly remove the woman by lifting her buttocks upward. The woman dismounts and either he or she squeezes the base of his penis, continuing non-demand coitus only when the man feels he is under control.

The idea is that the couple slowly work themselves up to penile thrusting, stopping as needed for the squeeze. The man can also periodically squeeze his penis at its base if necessary during intercourse. Although the squeeze does reduce the urgency to ejaculate, it can also cause a partial loss of erection. (See figure 9.5.)

❖ The stop-and-start method is just as it sounds. During intercourse, when a man feels he is close to ejaculating, he

Figure 9.5 Squeeze technique

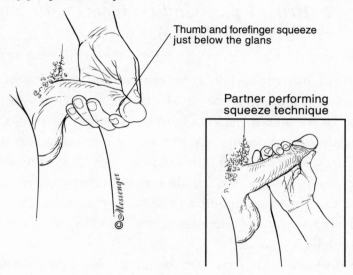

Thumb and forefinger squeeze just below the glans

Partner performing squeeze technique

©*Messenger*

stops and withdraws from his partner's vagina. When he feels he has regained control, he begins again. As he becomes desensitized, he may just need to stop and not withdraw. As with the squeeze technique, a cooperative and understanding partner is essential. It also helps to start with intercourse positions that provide the least amount of friction, such as side-by-side or facing each another.

Obviously, both techniques are often combined. But do they work? Early ejaculation is a difficult problem to treat, and overcoming it takes a lot of patience, practice, and self-control. It also takes time, perhaps months. The success rate in treating it is not as strong as with other disorders. Some doctors now say they can treat early ejaculation more successfully with antidepressants like Prozac, Zoloft, or Anafranil. (See chapter 7 for more information.)

How to Bring Up Sexual Problems with Your Doctor

First, remember that a doctor is human, too, and that he or she may have anxieties about discussing sexuality with patients. Don't take it personally or as a judgment on you if your doctor becomes uncomfortable. Although anatomy and physiology may have been thoroughly addressed in medical school, to the extent that female sexual anatomy is presently understood, courses on human sexuality or sexual history are relatively recent phenomena and not consistently addressed in all medical schools.

But second, don't take no for an answer. Some doctors may minimize your problem or dismiss it, but that's usually because they don't know how to help. They think it may be psychological, or they are not aware of any potential treatments. For these reasons, educating yourself and arming yourself with information to take to your doctor will be extremely helpful to him or her as well as to you. Most doctors are not trained to deal with sexual problems, and due to the limited amount of information in the literature at this time, fewer are aware of the cutting-edge research in this field. If your doctor avoids addressing your sexual problems, acknowledge that the subject is embarrassing for both of you, but make it clear that your sexuality is a basic part of you. Start the conversation on a positive note: "I was hoping that you might be able to help me with this problem I have."

Many women find that it helps to bring literature or an article with them to their doctor to start the conversation: "I was reading this and wondered what you thought." Or bring in this book!

Finally, be persistent. If you don't get the response you want, you should not feel bad about finding another physician. (See our Resources section at the end of this chapter.) Our goal is to help your physicians and health care providers help you reach your full sexual potential. Most doctors will be open and receptive to your comments and will be happy to learn of any new information you can provide. Quite possibly your doctor will have already encouraged you to look elsewhere, having exhausted his or her own resources. Unfortunately, all too often the first outside referral is to a therapist, assuming that the problem is completely psychological. Such was the history of male erectile dysfunction 20 years ago.

If you're having trouble finding a doctor willing to talk about sexual issues, you might try looking in your local yellow pages or checking with your local hospital for a recommendation of women's health center. Even if the center doesn't treat sexual function complaints themselves, they usually have a network of physicians who are sympathetic to women's issues.

How to Find a Good Sex Therapist

The American Association of Sex Educators, Counselors, and Therapists (AASECT) has lists of thousands of qualified sex therapists all over the United States. (See our Resources section at the end of this chapter.) You can call, write, or e-mail AASECT to find the names of sex therapists near you. If you send them a request with a stamped, self-addressed envelope, they will send you a list of certified sex therapists in your area. You can also contact your local licensing board of the American Psychological (or Psychiatric) Association or the National Association of Social Workers to find a general therapist. Once you have a list, you should be able to call different therapists in your area and ask them about their experience with your type of complaint, or you can meet with a therapist once on a trial basis to see if you feel comfortable.

In searching for a therapist, you should ideally be looking for someone who has credentials and experience as a sex therapist but who is also trained as a general therapist. That way the therapist can effectively attend to your sexual concerns but also to the larger emotional issues or relationship conflicts that may arise. If you need help with your partner, your therapist should also have experience with couples therapy. Therapists should be licensed, meaning that they have gone through the proper education, training, and licensing procedures. Licensing requires that therapists answer to regulatory boards that demand continuous education and competence, maintain quality control, and give you resources with which to act if you have a complaint or feel that you have been treated unethically.

Therapists can be clinical social workers, psychologists, or psychiatrists. It doesn't really matter as long as you're comfortable, although psychiatrists have medical degrees and are able to prescribe medication. It is perfectly acceptable for you to ask about your therapist's training, and whether the therapist has experience treating your specific problem. It is also acceptable to ask about fees.

Although sex therapy in and of itself is usually not covered by health insurance, it may be covered as a couples problem or under a broader diagnosis like depression, anxiety, or posttraumatic stress disorder, depending on the nature of the complaint. Every state and health plan is different. Educate yourself about what is available to you and confer with your therapist. Many therapists charge between $120 to $150 for a 45-minute to one-hour session, although some will adjust fees to your economic needs.

SEXUAL SELF-ASSESSMENT QUESTIONNAIRE

How to Determine if You Have a Sexual Problem, and if Medical Intervention Can Help

The following questionnaire is designed to help you start to determine if your problem is psychological, physiological, or a combination of the two. Clearly this questionnaire does not replace your doctor or therapist, but it may help point you in the right direction and put you in the right frame of mind for seeking help.

Have you been suffering with sexual function complaints such as vaginal dryness, decreased genital sensation, or difficulty achieving orgasm and are wondering if they might be due to a medical or physiologic problem? The following questions will give you some sense as to whether medical intervention may help. See page 222 for the answers and further explanation.

Answer yes to the statements you would agree with.

1. During sexual stimulation, foreplay, and/or intercourse, I experience the following sexual complaint(s): (check all that apply)
   a. vaginal dryness   Yes   No
   b. lack of genital sensation (tingling/ warmth with sexual arousal)   Yes   No
   c. difficulty achieving orgasm   Yes   No
   d. loss of intensity of orgasm (orgasms feel muffled)
                                                          Yes   No
   e. genital pain either with or without sexual contact
                                                          Yes   No
   f. lack of sexual interest   Yes   No

2. I feel that my sexual complaint(s) have affected my desire for sex. In other words, if sex wasn't painful, frustrating, or no fun, I would be more interested.
                                   Yes   No   Don't know

3. I notice that I have the same sexual difficulties with my partner as I have alone during self-stimulation.
   Yes   No   Don't know   Don't self-stimulate

4. There was a time when I was satisfied with my sexual response and/or interest.
                                   Yes   No   Don't know

5. I am presently being treated with medication and/or psychotherapy for:
   a. depression   Yes   No

 b. anxiety disorder   Yes   No
 c. any psychiatric illness   Yes   No

6. I feel that:
 a. My partner knows what to do to sexually satisfy me.
                Yes   No
 b. I am comfortable giving my partner direction about how to sexually stimulate me.   Yes   No
 c. I feel connected to and emotionally intimate with my partner.   Yes   No
 d. My general/sexual communication with my partner is adequate.   Yes   No
 e. I don't have a partner at present.   Yes   No

7. I have a history of sexual abuse or trauma.
          Yes   No   Don't know
 If yes,
 a. I never told anyone.   Yes   No
 b. I never pressed charges.   Yes   No
 c. I did not receive counseling.   Yes   No
 d. I feel this history affects my present sexual life.
                Yes   No

8. The following conditions apply to me:
 a. I have had a hysterectomy or other pelvic surgery.
                Yes   No
 b. I am postmenopausal.   Yes   No
 c. I have diabetes.   Yes   No
 d. I have cardiovascular disease.   Yes   No
 e. I smoke.   Yes   No
 f. I am taking SSRI's (such as Zoloft or Prozac).
                Yes   No
 g. I am taking birth control pills.   Yes   No

h. I have had one or more prolonged labor and deliveries (that is, needed ventuse/suction).   Yes   No

i. I have a history of straddle injury (fell on a bicycle, balance beam, etc.).   Yes   No

j. I have had a back injury and/or back surgery.

Yes   No

k. I have had a spinal chord injury.   Yes   No

l. I have had genital circumcision.   Yes   No

m. I have multiple sclerosis or other neurologic disorder.

Yes   No

Answers

1. If you answered yes to:

    1a and/or 1b: You have symptoms of female sexual arousal disorder (**FSAD**).

    1c and/or 1d: You have symptoms of female orgasmic disorder (**FOD**).

    1e: You have symptoms of sexual pain disorder.

    1f: You have symptoms of hypoactive desire disorder (**HDD**).

Now let's see if there are any clues about what kind of intervention might help.

2. If you answered yes, your hypoactive desire symptoms may be, in part, a result of your sexual arousal and/or sexual response. In other words, if sex is frustrating, painful, or no fun because of an arousal or response

problem, you may have lost your motivation. Treatment should be focused on those complaints as much as or more than your diminished desire. However, if loss of desire is your only complaint, then treatment should focus on this issue.

3. If you answered yes, this is an indication that your complaint may be medically based. If you answered no, you are certainly not alone. Many women find it difficult to reach orgasm with their partner, but have no problem achieving orgasm with self-stimulation. You may want to look into the possibility that there may be some other problems, such as stress in your relationship, playing a role in your sexual complaints.

4. If you answered yes, this is an indication that your complaint may be medically based. If you answered no, you have what is called a primary complaint, meaning it has always existed. There may be a medical basis to your complaint and you should seek a physician's help. At present, however, most medications and interventions are focused on women who were satisfied with their sexual response at one point in time but now because of organic or medical reasons no longer respond as they did. Perhaps we will continue to learn more about the physical components of what is called primary sexual function complaints. In the meantime, you may want to talk to your doctor about neurologic testing as well as the possibility of seeking support from a general or sex therapist.

5. If you answered yes, although there may be medical issues to consider, you might want to look into the possibility that your sexual complaints are related to your
   anxiety, depression, or other mental health concerns.

6. If you answered yes to 6a, 6b, 6c, and 6d, this is an indicator that your complaints may be more medically based
   than related to sexual communication problems in your
   relationship. If you answered no, then there may be issues or conflicts in your relationship that are contributing
   to your sexual complaints.

7. If you answered yes, and also answered yes to 7a, 7b, 7c,
   or 7d, you may want to look into the possibility that your
   sexual complaints could be related to this traumatic
   history.

8. If you answered yes to any of 8a through 8m, this is an
   indicator that your sexual complaints could be medically
   based. All of the listed conditions are medical risk factors
   for sexual dysfunction.

Now what do you do with these clues?

Obviously, you can't be evaluated or diagnosed for sexual
dysfunction and its sources exclusively on the basis of this
questionnaire. An evaluation in person is necessary. We hope
this has helped you with some initial clues for follow-up. You
have some choices about what to do.

If you want more information, or a fuller picture of what
might be at the root of your sexual complaints, you can
complete a more comprehensive questionnaire on-line

at www.newshe.com, the Web site for our Network for Excellence in Women's Sexual Health. Once we have your answers, you will receive a personalized report on-line about your sexual health that may be of use in understanding your problem and seeking appropriate treatment.

If you feel that there may be some relationship or emotional problems contributing, even if only in part, to your sexual function complaints, seek out the help of an individual, couples, or sex therapist. For this, see *How to Find a Good Sex Therapist*, page 217, or consult our Resources section below. Remember, it is the rare case that is purely physiological or purely emotional. Usually it is a combination of both components. Each piece of the puzzle needs to be addressed as it interacts with the others to provide lasting relief.

Resources

Compounding Pharmacies

There are thousands of them across the country. We use
Urgent Care Pharmacy
227 Winchester Place, Suite 106
Spartanburg, SC 29209
(800) 692-6982, Fax (888) 235-9350
www.urgentcarepharmacy.com, E-mail urgentcarepharmacy
@msn.com

The International Academy of Compounding Pharmacists
(IACP)
P.O. Box 1365
Sugar Land, TX 77487
(800) 927–4227, Fax (281) 495-0602
www.iacprx.org, E-mail iacpinfo@iacprx.org
Call or enter your zip code on the Web site for a list of compounding pharmacies in your area.

Disabilities

ABLED!
This is a newsletter for "active, beautiful, loving, exquisite, disabled women."
ABLED Publications
12211 Fondren, Suite 703
Houston, TX 77035
(713) 726-1132

The Center for Research on Women with Disabilities
(CROWD)
A research center that focuses on issues related to health, aging, civil rights, abuse, and independent living.
3440 Richmond Avenue, Suite B
Houston, TX 77046
(713) 960-0505, Toll Free (800) 44-CROWD, Fax (713) 961-3555
www.bcm.tmc.edu/crowd, E-mail crowd@bcm.tmc.edu

Project on Women and Disability
43 Waban Hill Road North
Newton, MA 02467
(617) 969-4974
Support groups, information, and referrals, research in all
areas of living with a disability

Resourceful Women: Women with Disabilities Striving toward Health and Self-Determination
The Health Resource Center for Women with Disabilities
publishes a free quarterly newsletter for women featuring
articles on sexual health and covering issues such as breast
cancer and disabled women's access to mammography and
resourceful parenting.
Rehabilitation Institute of Chicago
345 East Superior Street, Room 1562
Chicago, IL 60611
(800) 354-7342 or (312) 238-1055
www.rehabchicago.org, E-mail webmaster@rehabchicago.
org

The Sexual Health Network
3 Mayflower Lane
Huntington, CT 06484
(203) 924-4623
www.sexualhealth.com
Provides easy access to sexuality information, education,
counseling, therapy, medical attention, and other sexuality
resources for people with disability, illness, or other health related problems.

Enhancing Sexual Pleasure

There are numerous sexual aids available to enhance your sexual pleasure. For instance, there are good small vibrators to use with intercourse, such as the Pocket Rocket, or vibrators that your partner can strap on to his penis. Both stimulate the clitoris during genital penetration. These vibrators are relatively strong for their small size. Even stronger are the larger wand-style vibrators, commonly known as massagers. They are typically used either alone or with a partner, but are not easy to manipulate during intercourse. Regardless, there is a huge range of vibrators and other products to choose from.

We encourage women to visit an erotica shop in person, where they can see and handle the vibrators and get assistance. They can also mail order or order on-line if they don't have direct access, although the on-line stores typically only have a portion of the entire stock available. You can also find great books in these shops as well.

There are also instructional and erotic videos. Some can be obtained through the erotica shops mentioned below, specifically videos created by Candida Royalle at Femme Productions. She is an ex-erotica star who decided to start making videos by and for women that actually have a plot. Nina Hartley is also an erotica star who makes educational videos for women, men, and couples. Sinclaire Intimacy Institute at (800) 955-0888 or www.bettersex.com is a wonderful source for educational videos, including couples educational videos (for introducing new ideas to your partner), videos on sex and aging, and some general instructional videos as well.

Some of the best known female friendly resources are:

Betty Dodson Workshops
P.O. Box 1933
Murray Hill Station
New York, NY 10156
www.bettydodson.com
For excellent courses, videos, and books on self-stimulation
and self-loving. On-line discussion and advice on many sex-
related topics.

Eve's Garden International, Ltd.
119 W. 57 Street
New York, NY 10019
(800) 848-3837, Fax (781) 593-0487
www.evesgarden.com
On-line catalog offers a wide variety of sex toys, scented
massage oils, and other items, as well as a selection of educational and erotic books and videos for women and
couples.

Good Vibrations
1210 Valencia Street
San Francisco, CA 94110
(800) BUY-VIBE, (415) 974-8990
www.goodvibes.com, E-mail goodvibe@well.com
Founded by Joani Blank in 1977, this retail store and on-line
catalog specialize in vibrators, sex toys, and erotic books and
videos.

Grand Opening! Sexuality Boutique
318 Harvard Street, Suite 32
Brookline, MA 02446
(617) 731-2626, Fax (617) 731-2693
grandopening.com, E-mail office@grandopening.com

Marriage and Family Health Center
2922 Evergreen Parkway, Suite 310
Evergreen, CO 80439
(303) 670-2630, Fax (303) 670-2392
www.passionatemarriage.com
Founded by Dr. David Schnarch and Dr. Ruth Morehouse, for couples, relationship and sexuality enhancement courses, including Passionate Marriage couples retreats and couples enrichment weekends.

Tantra Workshops
c/o S. Wadel and D. Coleman
1470 DeHaro Street
San Francisco, CA 94107
For workshops in the tantric arts and Eastern approaches to sexuality.

Family Planning and Women's Health

The Network for Excellence in Women's Sexual Health
Newshe.com is our own Web site and network of clinics, dedicated to helping women find solutions for reaching their full sexual potential. On the site you'll find additional guidance, education, and support for women with sexual function complaints; treatment strategies; information and resources for professionals treating women; chat, bulletin boards, e-mail, interactive surveys, and a chance to tell your story. You will also find an extensive referral network for the growing number of physicians and therapists who are expanding into the field of women's sexual dysfunction.
www.newshe.com

Planned Parenthood Federation of America, Inc.
810 Seventh Avenue
New York, NY 10022
(212) 541-7800, (800) 230-PLAN, Fax (212) 245-1845
www.plannedparenthood.org
Planned Parenthood is the world's largest and oldest voluntary family planning organization. An excellent resource for
information about birth control, abortion, and women's
health.

National Alliance of Breast Cancer Organizations (NABCO)
1180 Avenue of the Americas, 2nd Floor
New York, NY 10036
(212) 221-3300
Financial assistance (medication, radiation, chemotherapy,
transport, home care, child care), counseling (in person or on
the phone), support groups (in person or on the phone), educational materials related to diagnosis and treatments. They have
a lot of information on sexuality and breast cancer as well.

National Women's Health Network
514 10 Street NW, Suite 400
Washington, DC 20004
general number: (202) 347-1140
information clearinghouse: (202) 628-7814
A women's health information clearinghouse, from which
they produce information packets and fact sheets on different women's health topics. They also attend to specific health
questions, researching answers, and providing resources to
women.

Interstitial Cystitis Association
51 Monroe Street, Suite 1402
Rockville, MD 20850
(800) HELP-ICA, (301) 610-5300, Fax (301) 610-5308
www.ichelp.org, E-mail:icamail@ichelp.org
A not-for-profit health organization dedicated to providing
patient and physician educational information and programs,
patient support, public awareness, and research funding.

National Vulvadynia Association
P.O. Box 4491
Silver Spring, MD 20914-4491
(301) 299-0775, Fax (301) 299-3999
www.nva.org

Vulvar Pain Foundation
203½ North Main Street, Suite 203
Graham, NC 27253
(336) 226-0704, Fax (336) 226-8518
www.vulvarpainfoundation.org

www.uterinefibroids.com
On-line resource developed by Carla Dionne, author of *Sex,
Lies, and Uterine Fibroids.*
e-mail carla@uterinefibroids.com

Lesbian Issues

GLOBAL (Gay and Lesbian Organizations Bridging across the Lands)
Greater San Diego Business Association (GSDBA)
P.O. Box 33848
San Diego, CA 92163
(619) 296-4543, Fax (619) 296-5616

gsdba.org/global.html
GLOBAL is a nonprofit international association of gay and lesbian organizations sharing a common goal of professional and personal enrichment.

Maternity and Childbirth

American College of Nurse-Midwives
818 Connecticut Avenue NW, Suite 900
Washington, DC 20006
(202) 728-9860, Fax (202) 728-9897
www.midwife.org, E-mail info@acnm.org
For information about contacting midwives trained in natural childbirth, prenatal and postnatal care, and maternal psychological issues.

Maternal Fitness
108 East 16 Street
New York, NY 10003
(212) 353-1947, Fax (212) 353-0620
www.maternalfitness.com, E-mail info@maternalfitness.com

Created by Julie Tupler, who wrote a book with the same name, *Maternal Fitness*, has prenatal training, exercise, and conditioning taught by registered nurses who are also personal trainers and are at the forefront of this trend.

Menopause

North American Menopause Society (NAMS)
5900 Landerbrook Drive, Suite 195
Mayfield Heights, OH 44124
(440) 442-7550, Fax (440) 442-2660
www.menopause.org, E-mail info@menopause.org
Automated Consumer Request Line (800) 774-5342

Seniors

The National Institute on Aging
Building 31, Room 5C27
31 Center Drive, MSC 2292
Bethesda, MD 20892
(301) 496-1752
www.nih.gov/nia

Sexual Abuse

VOICES in Action (Victims of Incest Can Emerge Survivors)
P.O. Box 148309
Chicago, IL 60614
(773) 327-1500, (800) 7-VOICE-8
voices-action.org

National network of incest survivors. They have more than 100 special interest support groups who correspond with each other in a systematic way.

The Healing Woman Foundation
P.O. Box 28040
San Jose, CA 95159
(408) 246-1788, Fax (520) 569-6141
www.healingwoman.org, E-mail HealingW@healingwoman.
org
Nonprofit organization dedicated to providing recovery resources for women survivors of childhood sexual abuse. They publish a bimonthly, 24-page (print only) newsletter covering all aspects of recovery, including advice from healing professionals as well as contributions from survivors themselves.

Sexuality Education and Therapy

American Association of Sex Educators, Counselors, and Therapists (AASECT)
P.O. Box 238
Mount Vernon, IA 53214-0238
(319) 895-8407, Fax (319) 895-6203
www.aasect.org, E-mail AASECT@worldnet.att.net
For information and referrals for certified sex therapists all over the country.

American Psychological Association
750 First Street NE
Washington, DC 20002-4242
(202) 336-5541
A good referral service for board-certified psychologists.

Sexuality Information and Education Council of the United
States (SIECUS)
West 42 Street, Suite 350
New York, NY 10036-7802
(212) 819-9770, Fax (212) 819-9776
www.siecus.org, E-mail siecus@siecus.org
SIECUS is a national nonprofit organization which affirms
that sexuality is a natural and healthy part of living. An excellent source, with an extensive library filled with information about sexuality and sex education.

Society for Human Sexuality
PMB 1276
1122 East Pike Street
Seattle, WA 98122-3934
www.sexuality.org, E-mail shs@sexuality.org
An organization devoted to the understanding and enjoyment of all safe and consensual forms of sexual expression.

Further Reading

Barbach, L. *The Pause: Positive Approaches to Menopause*. Penguin,
  1993.
Blank, Joani. *Good Vibrations: The Complete Guide to Vibrators*.
  Down There Press, 1989.

Boston Women's Health Collective. *Our Bodies, Ourselves for the New Century.* Simon & Schuster, 1998.

Chia, Mantak, and Maneewan Chia. *Healing Love through the Tao: Cultivating Female Sexual Energy.* Healing Tao Books, 1986.

Comfort, Alex. *The Joy of Sex.* Crown, 1972.

———. *More Joy: A Lovemaking Companion to "The Joy of Sex."* Crown, 1985.

———. *The New Joy of Sex.* Crown, 1991.

Dodson, Betty. *Sex for One: The Joy of Selfloving.* Crown, 1996.

Fisher, Helen. *Anatomy of Love: The Natural History of Monogamy, Adultery, and Divorce.* W. W. Norton, 1992.

———. *The First Sex: The Natural Talents of Women and How They Are Changing the World.* Random House, 1999.

———. *The Sex Contract: The Evolution of Human Behavior.* William Morrow, 1983.

Gross, Z. *Seasons of the Heart: Men and Women Talk about Love, Sex, and Romance after 60.* New World Library, 2000.

Heiman, Julia R., and Joseph LoPiccolo. *Becoming Orgasmic: A Sexual and Personal Growth Program for Women.* Prentice-Hall, 1988.

Hepburn, C., and B. Gutierrez, *Alive and Well: A Lesbian Health Guide.* Crossing Press, 1988.

Klein, E., and K. Kroll. *Enabling Romance: A Guide to Love, Sex, and Relationships for the Disabled.* Harmony Books, 1999.

Loulan, J. *Lesbian Sex.* Book People, 1984.

Maxfield, G., and Fannie Toner (eds.). *The Novel Approach to Sexuality and Disability.* Northern Nevada Amputee Support Group, 1996.

Ogden, G. *Women Who Love Sex.* Pocket Books, 1994.

Rako, Susan. *The Hormone of Desire: The Truth about Testosterone, Sexuality, and Menopause.* Three Rivers Press, 1999.

Schnarch, David, Ph.D. *Passionate Marriage.* Owl Books,
1998.
Shakespeare, T., K. Gillespie-Sells, and D. Davies. *The Sexual
Politics of Disability: Untold Desires.* Cassel Academic, 1996.
Shandler, Nina. *Estrogen: The Natural Way.* Villard Books,
1998.
Tupler, Julie, and Andrea Thompson. *Maternal Fitness:
Preparing for the Marathon of Labor.* Fireside, 1996.
Villarosa, L. (ed.). *Body and Soul: The Black Women's Guide to
Physical Health and Emotional Well-Being.* HarperCollins, 1994.
Winks, C. and A. Seamans. *The New Good Vibrations Guide to
Sex.* Cleis Press, 1997.
Zolbrod, Aline P. *Sex Smart: How Your Childhood Shaped Your
Sexual Life and What to Do about It.* Oakland, Calif.: New
Harbinger Publications, 1998.

Journals

Annual Review of Sex Research. Society for the Scientific Study
of Sexuality, Box 208, Mt. Vernon, IA 52314-0208.
Journal of Homosexuality. The Haworth Press, Inc., 10 Alice
St., Binghamton, NY 13904-1580.
Journal of Sex Education and Therapy. American Association of
Sex Educators, Counselors, and Therapists (AASECT),
Box 208, Mt. Vernon, IA 52314-0208.
Journal of Sex Research. Society for the Scientific Study of
Sexuality, Box 208, Mt. Vernon, IA 52314-0208.
Sexuality and Disability. Human Sciences Press, Inc., 233
Spring St., New York, NY 10013-1578.
SIECUS Reports. Sexuality Information and Education Council
of the United States, 130 West 42 Street, Suite 2500, New
York, NY 10036.

CHAPTER TEN

The Future

In the few years since we opened the Women's Sexual Health Clinic, the study and treatment of female sexual dysfunction has accelerated at a speed we never imagined. New studies and potential treatments evolve on an almost weekly basis. Pharmaceutical companies are racing to develop blood-flow–enhancing agents and testosterone supplements designed solely for women. Other companies are developing topical drugs and natural herbal and botanical products to treat female sexual complaints. However, few, if any, of these treatments will work without therapeutic support.

Doctors around the country have ceased trying to define female sexual dysfunction as "female impotence." They are ever more aware of the sexual problems of women and contact us almost daily to exchange information. The media has certainly helped feed the new awareness. Articles now appear regularly in newspapers, magazines, and journals about new breakthroughs, research, and attitudes, stimulating interest in male as well as female readers. Medical journals are incorporating FSD studies and FSD review articles into their monthly issues, and the number of researchers in this field is steadily growing.

We are enormously encouraged by what we see. Most gratifying of all, more women are beginning to feel comfortable seeking treatment for sexual complaints and are learning that sexual problems are not just "in their heads" but are recognized and treatable medical disorders.

We foresee big changes over the next decade as information and interest continue to evolve among patients, therapists, and physicians. We fully expect that hospitals will develop departments of sexual medicine, staffed by multidisciplinary teams of urologists, gynecologists, endocrinologists, colon and rectal surgeons, general practitioners, psychiatrists, psychotherapists, sex therapists, and others. The goal, like ours, will be to treat the whole woman, to include the physical and emotional causes for sexual dysfunction, as they are often related and feed on one another.

Having completed our work at Boston University, we are now establishing a major center for women's urology and sexual health called the Center for Pelvic Medicine at UCLA in Los Angeles in conjunction with Dr. Schlomo Raz and the UCLA Department of Urology. The center will focus on all urogenital and sexual health problems in women, including hormone deficiencies, pelvic floor problems, urinary and bladder problems, emotional problems and more. When women visit our center, they can expect a full sexual health checkup, something we hope will be routine at all doctors' offices in the future. We expect that the best forms and dosages of testosterone will soon be developed, making testosterone supplements for women as regulated and accepted as estrogen is now. We continue to believe that testosterone is extremely important in governing not only libido but also sexual response. The impact of testosterone on the central nervous system, in particular the brain, will be determined, providing explanations for the cyclical changes women experience in their libido and arousal during the menstrual cycle and throughout their lives.

We also hope to see more research into the loss of female libido after childbirth, which we suspect may be related to long-term testosterone or enzyme deficiencies not yet fully understood. We also hope to learn the mechanisms underlying the orgasmic response, what enhances and diminishes it, why some women are able to have multiple orgasms and others are not, and what pharmacological agents may be useful in women with orgasmic disorder.

Viagra, the drug that treats erectile dysfunction in men and has in many ways helped spur the interest in the sexual lives of women, will likely be approved for use by women by the Food and Drug Administration in the next several years. Viagra will remain a good treatment for some women, but there are also promising Viagra competitors that will be on the market within the next several years. Numerous herbal remedies, like yohimbine, have potential, too. It is important to realize that both medical and herbal remedies may have significant side effects, which should be appreciated prior to their use.

Perhaps the most critical need for the future is to develop a thorough understanding of the nerve supply to the female genitalia and pelvis in order to fully understand the physiologic and neurologic mechanisms for sexual arousal as well as genital pain. In particular, what nerves are responsible for vaginal sensation and uterine contractions during orgasm? What causes the burning, sharp, nerve-related pain in women with vulvadynia? And why do some women experience loss of vaginal and clitoral sensation following hysterectomy?

The development of nerve-sparing pelvic surgery for women, similar to what was developed in the 1970s for men, is essential. We continue to believe that injury to nerves and small arterial branches supplying blood to the uterus and vagina during pelvic surgery has the potential for causing sexual function problems. There is much research currently under way, such as cadaver studies tracing the nerves to the uterus, vagina, and clitoris. In the operating room, nerve stimulation techniques are helping surgeons understand the nerve distribution in the pelvic area. Since vessels and nerves often run together, a vascular benefit will likely accompany efforts at increasing nerve preservation in pelvic surgeries. Over the next year we hope we will begin to put some pieces of the puzzle together.

There is still much to learn about the sexual anatomy of women. As it stands now, we are only beginning to understand the complex mechanisms behind female sexual function and response. We know where the sensory and motor nerves are throughout the body, and we know what occurs physiologically as the sexual organs respond to impulses from the brain. But nobody has been able to describe the exact nerve pathways governing vaginal sensation and arousal. Our central nervous system is far more involved in sexual response than we presently understand—not only in women, but also in men. Almost certainly, the current explosion of research into women's sexual function will help solve problems in male sexuality as well.

People often ask us how sex will change in the new millennium. The most obvious development brought on by the technology boom has been the availability of sex on the Internet and the use of cybersex, or chatting on-line erotically, to connect to other people. Positive aspects of cybersex are that it's an optimal form of safer sex, it's a good way to be involved with partners long distance, and it's helpful for shy or intimidated people who may have a difficult time meeting people, especially sexual partners, or even expressing themselves sexually. There are also some creative new forms of cybersex under design, particularly Vivid Entertainment's "cybersex suit" for both men and women. The suit will wire into your computer and allow your cybersex partner to stimulate your different erogenous zones with a click of a mouse.

There are a number of downsides to cybersex. Clearly it can encourage a person to take on different personal and sexual identities and perhaps become so dependent on fantasy relationships that real life relationships can't develop. Although cybersex is exciting as an alternative, it also reflects our impatience and desire for a quick fix, often at the expense of intimacy. We will surely see the increasing impact of this phenomenon on individuals and couples in coming years, both in extramarital cyberrelationships, intimacy problems, social avoidance, and cybersex addiction.

We'll also see a trend in the new millennium toward what we call "serial monogamy." In other words, as people live longer, choosing one mate for life may not always be a realistic option. Because of the technological and medical breakthroughs expected in the next decade, many doctors believe that if you're alive in the year 2010 you may well live into your 100s. Marriages that once lasted a maximum of 30, 40, or 50 years could last 80 or more years. Some people may choose to become involved with partners for shorter periods of time. Interestingly, divorce rates in the United States are now stable, at about 50 percent, but remarriage rates are on the rise—a positive sign, we think, that there is less shame about failed marriages and that greater risks are being taken at giving love and intimacy and commitment a second chance. It also suggests that serial monogamy may already be on the rise.

We plan to continue to expand the pathways that we have helped define so far, and to help as many women as possible to achieve better understanding of their sexuality and greater sexual satisfaction. As an adjunct to our clinical efforts, we have formed the Network for Excellence in Women's Sexual Health, or NEWSHE, an organization dedicated to furthering research, information, and education in this field. Through our Web site, www.newshe.com, we hope to become a vital resource not only for women and their partners, but for the physicians, therapists, nurses, and other health professionals who treat them. We anticipate that both patients and physicians can use this service for referrals and for information about training and research. We also plan to have available through the Web site the NEWSHE sexual self-assessment questionnaire (an abridged version is provided here in chapter 9), which can help you determine if you have a sexual problem, the nature of the problem, and how you can find help. Women who are trying to get a sense of the roots of their problem will be able to fill out the questionnaire on-line, then receive a computer-generated report of their results. Our Web site will also have information about the NEWSHE foundation, a nonprofit organization created to further research in women's sexual health and to provide grants to researchers seeking answers.

One troubling aspect is the ongoing attitude of many doctors, women as well as men, to female sexual dysfunction. Laura recently conducted an on-line survey asking women about their experiences seeking help from their physicians for sexual problems. Although the survey may well have attracted a self-selecting group of women who wanted to air complaints, 42 percent said that their physicians were reluctant to help them. More than half said they felt frustration or anxiety from their experience seeking medical help. Clearly, doctors will have to change as more women become aware of what's available and learn to expect, and demand, better treatment.

One positive change we've seen in the last year is that some doctors in the United States are now offering versions of our physiological sexual health testing, which we described in chapter 1. This is a welcome development. We hope that the use of this and other objective testing continues and keeps pace with the rapid advances in technology. In the meantime, many professionals in our field, both physicians and therapists, are working hard to develop standards of professional care for women with sexual function complaints. We intend our Web site to be a resource as the information evolves.

One important warning: although we are a long way from the orgasmatron in the Woody Allen movie *Sleeper*— you may remember that it was the satirical, futuristic walk-in chamber that produced an orgasm in a few seconds flat—the danger remains that the new drugs and devices will make sex too goal-oriented and too focused on intercourse and orgasm. As we've said many times throughout this book, sex— real sex—will always be about connecting with yourself and another person, knowing your body and your sexual needs, sharing yourself, and building intimacy with another human being. None of this is dependent on intercourse and orgasm.

Although we can't yet say that the field of women's sexual health is about to catch up with that of men, we can say that women are increasingly deciding that they deserve the same treatment as men. And once women truly feel entitled to their sexuality, they'll feel entitled to anything.

Bibliography

All case studies come from our practice and from interviews with our patients conducted between December 1998 and July 2000.

Introduction

Laumann, E. O., A. Paik, and R. C. Rosen. "Sexual Dysfunction in the United States: Prevalence and Predictors." *Journal of the American Medical Association* 281 (1999): 537–44.

Masters, William H., and Virginia E. Johnson. *Human Sexual Response.* Boston: Little, Brown, 1966.

Masters, William H., Virginia E. Johnson, and Robert C. Kolodny. *Human Sexuality.* New York: HarperCollins, 1992.

O'Connell, H. E., J. M. Hutson, C. R. Anderson, and R. J. Plenter. "Anatomical Relationship between Urethra and Clitoris." *Journal of Urology* 159 (1998): 1892–7.

Park, K., I. Goldstein, C. Andry, M. B. Siroky, R. J. Krane, and K. M. Azadzoi, "Vasculogenic Female Sexual Dysfunction: The Hemodynamic Basis for Vaginal Engorgement Insufficiency and Clitoral Erectile Insufficiency." *International Journal of Impotence Research* 1 (1997): 27–37.

Thakar, R., I. Manyonda, S. L. Stanton, P. Clarkson, and G. Robinson. "Bladder, Bowel and Sexual Function after Hysterectomy for Benign Conditions." *British Journal of Obstetrics and Gynecology* 104 (1997): 983–87.

Chapter One

Basson, R., R. McInnes, M. D. Smith, G. Hodgson, T. Spain, and N. Koppiker. "Efficacy and Safety of Sildenafil in Estrogenized Women with Sexual Dysfunction Associated with Female Sexual Arousal Disorder." *Obstetrics and Gynecology* 95 (2000) 4 Suppl. 1: S54.

Berman, J. R., L. A. Berman, T. J. Werbin, E. E. Flaherty, N. M. Leahy, and I. Goldstein, "Clinical Evaluation of Female Sexual Function: Effects of Age and Estrogen Status on Subjective and Physiologic Sexual Responses. *International Journal of Impotence Research* 11 (1999): Suppl. 1: 31–38.

Berman, J. R., L. A. Berman, T. J. Werbin, N. Leary, E. Flaherty, T. Chai, and I. Goldstein. "Effect of Sildenafil on Subjective and Physiologic Parameters of the Female Sexual Response in Women with Sexual Arousal Disorder." (Manuscript under publication.) Boston University Medical Center and University of Maryland Medical Center Departments of Urology.

Berman, J. R., and I. Goldstein. "Sildenafil in Postmenopausal Women with Sexual Dysfunction." *Urology* 54 (1999): 578–79.

Dodson, Betty. "Selfloving: Portrait of a Women's Sexuality Seminar." VHS format video.

Goldstein, I., and J. R. Berman. "Vasculogenic Female Sexual Dysfunction: Vaginal Engorgement and Clitoral Erectile Insufficiency Syndromes." *International Journal of Impotence Research* 10 (1998) Suppl. 2: S84–90.

Rhodes, J. C., K. H. Kjerulff, P. W. Langenberg, and G. M. Guzinski, "Hysterectomy and Sexual Functioning." *Journal of the American Medical Association* 282 (1999): 1934–41.

Chapter Two

Bumiller, Elisabeth. *May You Be the Mother of a Hundred Sons: A Journey among the Women of India.* New York: Random House, 1990.

Chesler, Ellen. *A Woman of Valor: Margaret Sanger and the Birth Control Movement in America.* New York: Simon & Schuster, 1992.

Dastur, R. H. *Sex Power: The Conquest of Sexual Inadequacy.* Bombay: IBH Publishing Co., 1983.

Bibliography

D'Emilio, John, and Estelle B. Freedman. *Intimate Matters: A History of Sexuality in America*. New York: Harper & Row, 1988.

Ellis, Havelock. *Studies in the Psychology of Sex*. New York: Random House, 1936.

Freud, Sigmund. "Formulations Regarding Two Principles in Mental Functioning." In *Selected Papers* 4: 13–21. London: Hogarth Press, 1946.

———. *A General Introduction to Psychoanalysis*. Garden City, N.Y.: Garden City Publishing, 1943.

———. *The Interpretation of Dreams*. James Strachey (ed.). New York: William Morrow, 1976.

Gay, Peter. "Education of the Senses." *Victoria to Freud*. (The Bourgeois Experience, Vol. 1) New York: Oxford University Press, 1984.

Kinsey, Alfred, et al. *Sexual Behavior in the Human Female*. Philadelphia: W. B. Saunders, 1953.

———. *Sexual Behavior in the Human Male*. Philadelphia: W. B. Saunders, 1948.

Koedt, Anne, Ellen Levine, and Anita Rapone. *Radical Feminism*. New York: Quadrangle Books, 1973.

Maines, Rachel P. *The Technology of Orgasm*. Baltimore: The Johns Hopkins University Press, 1999.

Masters, William H., Virginia E. Johnson, and Robert C. Kolodny. *Human Sexuality*. New York: HarperCollins, 1992.

Tannahill, Reay. *Sex in History*. New York: Stein & Day, 1980.

Chapter Three

Allison, Kathleen Cahill. *American Medical Association Complete Guide to Women's Health*, Ramona I. Slupik (ed.). New York: Random House, 1996.

Basson, R. "The Female Sexual Response: A Different Model." *Journal of Sex and Marital Therapy* 26 (2000): 51–65.

The Boston Women's Health Collective. *Our Bodies, Ourselves for the New Century*. New York: Simon & Schuster, 1998.

Ellison, Carol Rinkleib. *Women's Sexualities: Generations of Women Share Intimate Secrets of Sexual Self-Acceptance*. Oakland, Calif.: New Harbinger Publications, 2000.

Bibliography

Federation of Feminists Women's Health Centers. *A New View of a Woman's Body*. New York: Simon & Schuster, 1981.

Kaplan, Helen Singer. *Disorders of Sexual Desire and Other New Concepts and Techniques in Sex Therapy*. Philadelphia: Brunner-Mazel, 1979.

———. *The New Sex Therapy: Active Treatment of Sexual Dysfunctions*. New York: Random House, 1974.

Ladas, Alice Kahn, Beverly Whipple, and John D. Perry. *The G Spot and Other Recent Discoveries about Human Sexuality*. New York: Holt, Rinehart, and Winston, 1982.

Levin, R. J. "The Mechanisms of Human Female Arousal." *Annual Review of Sex Research* 3 (1992): 1–48.

———. "Sex and the Human Female Reproductive Tract—What Really Happens during and after Coitus." *International Journal of Impotence Research* 10 (1998), Suppl. 1: S14–21.

Masters, William H., Virginia E. Johnson, and Robert C. Kolodny. *Human Sexuality*. New York: HarperCollins, 1992.

O'Connell, H. E., J. M. Hutson, C. R. Anderson, and R. J. Plenter. "Anatomical Relationship between Urethra and Clitoris." *Journal of Urology* 159 (1998): 1892–97.

Chapter Four

Allison, Kathleen Cahill. *American Medical Association Complete Guide to Women's Health*, Ramona I. Slupik (ed.). New York: Random House, 1996.

Basson, R., J. Berman, A. Burnett, L. Derogatis, D. Ferguson, J. Fourcroy, I. Goldstein, A. Graziottini, J. Heiman, E. Laan, S. Leiblum, H. Padma-Nathan, R. Rosen, K. Segraves, R. T. Segraves, R. Shabsigh, G. Wagner, and B. Whipple. "Report of the International Consensus Development Conference on Female Sexual Dysfunction: Definitions and Classifications." *Journal of Urology* 163 (2000): 889–93.

Berman, J. R., L. A. Berman, T. J. Werbin, and I. Goldstein. "Female Sexual Dysfunction: Anatomy, Physiology, Evaluation and Treatment Options." *Current Opinion Urology* 9 (1999): 563–68.

Berman, J. R., M. R. Santos, and I. Goldstein. "Relationship between

Cardiovascular Risk Factors and Female Sexual Arousal Disorder."
Menopause Review: Menopause and Sexuality, 4 (4) (1999): 43–47.

Berman, L. A., J. R. Berman, S. Keane, T. Werbin, S. Chhabra, and I. Goldstein. "Hysterectomy and Sexual Function: A Role for Sildenafil?" Division of Urology, Boston University Medical Center. Presented at the Female Sexual Function Forum meetings, Boston, Mass., October 2000.

Blank, Joani, ed., photographs by Tee A. Corinne. *Femalia*. San Francisco: Down There Press, 1993.

Dodson, Betty. *Sex for One: The Joy of Selfloving*. New York: Crown, 1996.

The Boston Women's Health Collective. *The New Our Bodies, Ourselves*. New York: Simon & Schuster, 1984.

Graedon, Joe, and Teresa Graedon. *The People's Pharmacy*. New York: St. Martin's Griffin, 1996.

Lai, L. D., S. C. Goodwin, S. M. Bonilla, A. P. Lai, T. Yegul, S. Vott, and M. DeLeon, "Sexual Dysfunction after Uterine Artery Embolization." *Journal of Vascular and Interventional Radiology* (June 2000): 755–58.

LaSalle, M. D. "Bicycle Riding and Female Sexual Dysfunction." Boston University Medical Center Department of Urology. Presented at "New Perspectives in the Management of Female Dysfunction," October 23–25, 1998.

Masters, William H., Virginia E. Johnson, and Robert C. Kolodny. *Human Sexuality*. New York: HarperCollins, 1992.

Saunders Drug Handbook for Health Professionals 2000. Philadelphia: W. B. Saunders, 2000.

Schnarch, David Morris. *Passionate Marriage: Love, Sex, and Intimacy in Emotionally Committed Relationships*. New York: Norton, 1997.

Sipski, M. L., and C. J. Alexander. "Sexual Activities, Response and Satisfaction in Women Pre- and Post-Spinal Cord Injury." *Archives of Physical Medicine and Rehabilitation* 74 (1993): 1025–29.

Sipski, M. L., R. C. Rosen, C. J. Alexander, and R. M. Hamer. "Sildenafil Effects on Sexual and Cardiovascular Responses in Women with Spinal Cord Injury." *Urology* 55 (2000): 812–15.

Whipple, B., C. A. Gerdes, B. R. Komisaruk. "Sexual Response to Self-Stimulation in Women with Complete Spinal Cord Injury." *Journal of Sex Research* 33 (1996): 231–40.

Chapter Five

Berman, L. A., and J. R. Berman. "Viagra and Beyond: Where Sex Educators and Therapists Fit in from a Multi-Disciplinary Perspective." *Journal of Sex Education and Therapy*, 25 (1) (2000): 6.

Berman, J. R., L. A. Berman, T. J. Werbin, N. Leary, E. Flaherty, T. Chai, and I. Goldstein. "Effect of Sildenafil on Subjective and Physiologic Parameters of the Female Sexual Response in Women with Sexual Arousal Disorder." (Manuscript in press.) *Journal of Sex and Marital Therapy*.

Brody, Jane E. "Behind the Hoopla over a Hormone." *New York Times*, February 3, 1998, F8.

———. "Drug Researchers Working to Design Customized Estrogen." *New York Times*, March 4, 1997, C1.

———. "Hormone Replacement: Weighing Risks and Benefits." *New York Times*, February 1, 2000, F1.

Colditz, G. A., S. E. Hankinson, D. J. Hunter, W. C. Willett, J. E. Manson, M. J. Stampfer, C. Hennekens, B. Rosner, and F. E. Speizer, "The Use of Estrogens and Progestins and the Risk of Breast Cancer in Post-Menopausal Women." *New England Journal of Medicine* 332 (1995): 1589–93.

Cummings, S. R., S. Eckert, K. A. Krueger, D. Grady, T. J. Powles, J. A. Cauley, L. Norton, T. Nickelson, N. H. Bjarnason, M. Morrow, M. E. Lippman, D. Black, J. E. Glusman, A. Costa, and V. C. Jordan. "The Effect of Raloxifene on Risk of Breast Cancer in Postmenopausal Women: Results from the MORE Randomized Trial." *Journal of the American Medical Association* 281 (1999): 2189–97.

Greendale, G. A., N. P. Lee, and E. R. Arriola. "The Menopause." *Lancet* 353 (1999): 571–80.

Henig, Robin Marantz. "Behind the Buzz on Designer Estrogens, Questions Linger." *New York Times*, June 21, 1998. Sec. 15, 4.

Hermann, H. C., G. Chang, B. D. Klugherz, and P. D. Mahoney.

"Hemodynamic Effects of Sildenafil in Men with Severe Coronary Artery Disease." *New England Journal of Medicine* 342 (June 1, 2000)(22).

Hitt, Jack. "The Search for the Female Viagra and Other Tales from the Second Sexual Revolution." *New York Times Magazine*, February 20, 2000, 34–41, 50, 62, 64, 68–69.

Hulley, S., D. Grady, T. Bush, C. Furberg, D. Herrington, B. Riggs, and E. Vittinghoff. "Randomized Trial of Estrogen Plus Progestin for Secondary Prevention of Coronary Heart Disease in Post-Menopausal Women. Heart and Estrogen/Progestin Replacement Study (HERS) Research Group." *Journal of the American Medical Association* 280 (1998): 603–13.

Kolata, Gina. "Estrogen Tied to Slight Increase in Risks to Heart, a Study Hints." *New York Times*, April 5, 2000, A1.

———. "Ideas and Trends: Drugs That Deliver More Than Originally Promised." *New York Times*, April 5, 1998, Sec. 4, 3.

———. "U.S. Approves Sale of Impotence Pill; Huge Market Seen." *New York Times*, March 28, 1998, A1.

Meston, C. M. and M. Worcel. "The Effects of L-Arginine and Yohimbine on Sexual Arousal in Postmenopausal Women with FSAD." Department of Psychology, University of Texas at Austin; NitroMed, Inc., Bedford, Mass., 2000.

Rako, Susan. *The Hormone of Desire: The Truth about Testosterone, Sexuality, and Menopause.* Three Rivers Press, 1999.

Ross, J. K., A. Paganini-Hill, P. C. Wan, and M. C. Pike. "Effect of Hormone Replacement Therapy on Breast Cancer Risk: Estrogen versus Estrogen Plus Progestin." *Journal of the National Cancer Institute* 92 (2000): 328–32.

Rubio, E. A., M. Lopez, M. Lipezker, C. Rampazzo, M. T. Hurtado de Mendoza, F. Lowrey, L. A. Loehr, P. I. Lammers. "Evaluation of the Effects of Phentolamine Mesylate on Vaginal Blood Flow Response in Postmenopausal Women with Female Sexual Dysfunction." XVI FIGO World Congress of Gynecology and Obstetrics, Washington, D.C., September 7, 2000.

Schairer, C., J. Lubin, R. Troisi, S. Sturgeon, L. Brinton, and R. Hoover. "Menopausal Estrogen and Estrogen-Progestin Replacement Therapy and Breast Cancer Risk." *Journal of the American Medical Association* 283 (2000): 485–91.

Shandler, Nina. *Estrogen: The Natural Way: Over 250 Easy and Delicious Recipes for Menopause*. New York: Random House, 1998.

Shifren, J. L., G. D. Braunstein, J. A. Simon, P. R. Casson, J. E. Buster, G. P. Redmond, R. E. Burki, E. S. Ginsburg, R. C. Rosen, S. R. Leiblum, K. P. Jones, C. A. Daugherty, K. E. Caramelli, and N. A. Mazer. "Transdermal Testosterone Treatment in Women with Impaired Sexual Function after Oophorectomy." *New England Journal of Medicine* 343 (2000): 682–88.

Stanford, J. L., N. S. Weiss, L. F. Voight, J. R. Daling, L. A. Habel, and M. A. Rossing. "Combined Estrogen and Progestin Hormone Replacement Therapy in Relation to Risk of Breast Cancer in Middle-Aged Women." *Journal of the American Medical Association* 274 (1995): 137–42.

Walsh, Patrick C., and Janet Farrar Worthington. *The Prostate: A Guide for Men and the Women Who Love Them*. New York: Warner Books, 1997.

Chapter Six

Allison, Kathleen Cahill. *American Medical Association Complete Guide to Women's Health*, Ramona I. Slupik (ed.). New York: Random House, 1996.

The Boston Women's Health Collective. *Our Bodies, Ourselves for the New Century*. New York: Simon & Schuster, 1998.

Bouris, Karen. *The First Time: What Parents and Teenage Girls Should Know about "Losing Your Virginity."* Berkeley, Calif.: Conari Press, 1995.

Brody, Jane E. "Personal Health: Yesterday's Precocious Puberty is Norm Today." *New York Times*, November 30, 1999. F8.

Fisher, Helen. *Anatomy of Love: The Natural History of Monography, Adultery, and Divorce*. New York: W. W. Norton, 1992.

Fleming, J. M. "Prevalence of Childhood Sexual Abuse in a Community Sample of Australian Women." *Medical Journal of Australia* 166 (1997): 65–68.

Herman-Giddens, M. E., E. J. Slora, R. C. Wasserman, C. J. Bourdony, M. V. Bhapkar, G. G. Koch, and C. M. Hasemeier. "Secondary Sexual Characteristics and Menses in Young Girls

Seen in Office Practice: A Study from the Pediatric Research in Office Settings Network." *Pediatrics* 99 (1997): 505–12.

Kaplowitz, P. B., and S. E. Oberfield. "Re-examination of the Age Limit for Defining When Puberty Is Precocious in Girls in the United States: Implications for Evaluation and Treatment." *Pediatrics* 104 (1999): 936–41.

Kitzinger, Sheila. *Woman's Experience of Sex: The Facts and Feelings of Female Sexuality at Every Stage of Life*. New York: Penguin Books, 1985.

Masters, William H., Virginia E. Johnson, and Robert C. Kolodny. *Human Sexuality*. New York: HarperCollins, 1992.

Michael, Robert T., Edward O. Laumann, Gina Kolata, and John H. Gagnon. *Sex in America: A Definitive Survey*. New York: Little, Brown, 1995.

National Survey of Family Growth. National Center for Health Statistics, 1995.

National Survey of Family Growth. National Center for Health Statistics, 1990.

Stock, Jacqueline L., Michelle A. Bell, Debra K. Boyer, and Frederick A. Connell. "Adolescent Pregnancy and Sexual Risk-Taking among Sexually Abused Girls." *Family Planning Perspectives* (August/September 1997): 200–3, 227.

Zolbrod, Aline P. *Sex Smart: How Your Childhood Shaped Your Sexual Life and What to Do about It*. Oakland, Calif.: New Harbinger Publications, 1998.

Chapter Seven

Altman, Lawrence K., M.D. "The Doctor's World; Exploring the Enigma of Prostate Therapies." *New York Times*, May 9, 2000. F 8.

Carson, Culley C., Irwin Goldstein, and Roger S. Kirby. *Textbook of Erectile Dysfunction*. Isis Medical Media, 1999.

Krane, Robert J., Irwin Goldstein, and Mike B. Siroky. *Male Sexual Dysfunction*. New York: Little, Brown, 1983.

Moglia, Ronald Filiberti, Ed.D., and Jon Knowles (eds.). *Planned*

Parenthood All About Sex: A Family Resource on Sex and Sexuality. New York: Three Rivers Press, 1997.

Walsh, Patrick C., and Janet Farrar Worthington. *The Prostate: A Guide for Men and the Women Who Love Them.* New York: Warner Books, 1997.

Chapter Eight

Allison, Kathleen Cahill. *American Medical Association Complete Guide to Women's Health,* Ramona I. Slupik (ed.). New York: Random House, 1996.

The Boston Women's Health Collective. *Our Bodies, Ourselves for the New Century.* New York: Simon & Schuster, 1998.

Davey Smith, G., S. Frankel, and J. Yarnell. "Sex and Death: Are They Related? Findings from the Caerphilly Cohort Study." *British Medical Journal* 315 (1997): 1641–44.

Dionne, Carla. *www.uterinefibroids.com.*

Derby C. A., B. A. Mohr, I. Goldstein, H. A. Feldman, C. B. Johannes, and J. B. McKinlay. "Modifiable Risk Factors and Erectile Dysfunction: Can Lifestyle Changes Modify Risk?" *Urology* 56 (2000): 302–6.

Meston, C. M., and B. B. Gorzalka. "The Effects of Sympathetic Activation on Physiological and Subjective Sexual Arousal in Women." *Behavioral Research and Therapy* 33 (1995): 651–64.

Palmore, E. B. "Predictors of the Longevity Difference: A 25-Year Follow-Up." *Gerontologist* 22 (1982): 513–8.

Roizen, Michael F., M.D., with Elizabeth Anne Stephenson. *Real Age: Are You as Young as You Can Be?* New York: Cliff Street Books/ HarperCollins, 1999.

Chapter Nine

Allison, Kathleen Cahill. *American Medical Association Complete Guide to Women's Health,* Ramona I. Slupik (ed.). New York: Random House, 1996.

Eichel, Edward, and Philip Nobile. *The Perfect Fit: How to Achieve Mutual Fulfillment and Monogamous Passion through the New Intercourse.* New York: Donald I. Fine, 1992.

Bibliography

Eichel, E. W., J. D. Eichel, and S. Kule. "The Technique of Coital Alignment and Its Relation to Female Orgasmic Response and Simultaneous Orgasm." *Journal of Sex and Marital Therapy* 14 (1988): 129–141.

Heiman, Julia R., Ph.D., and Joseph LoPiccolo, Ph.D. *Becoming Orgasmic: A Sexual and Personal Growth Program for Women*. New York: Fireside, 1992.

Kaplan, Helen Singer. *The New Sex Therapy: Active Treatment of Sexual Dysfunctions*. New York: Random House, 1974.

Masters, William H., Virginia E. Johnson, and Robert C. Kolodny. *Human Sexuality*. New York: HarperCollins, 1992.

Moglia, Ronald Filiberti, Ed.D., and Jon Knowles (eds.). *Planned Parenthood All About Sex: A Family Resource on Sex and Sexuality*. New York: Three Rivers Press, 1997.

Pierce, A. P. "The Coital Alignment Technique (CAT): An Overview of Studies." *Journal of Sex and Marital Therapy* 26 (2000): 257–68.

Spencer, Amy. "New Sex Accelerator: His and Her Pleasure Triggers." *Glamour*, July 2000, 100–105.

Chapter Ten

Berman, Laura. "Patient Experience Survey." Network for Excellence in Women's Sexual Health, 2000, www.newshe.com.

Acknowledgments

There are many people to thank, without whom this book would not be possible. First and foremost, thank you to Elisabeth Bumiller who so eloquently put our thoughts and ideas into words; Binky Urban, our agent, for her phenomenal insights, advice, and advocacy; at Henry Holt and Company, Elizabeth Stein, for her talents as an editor, her patience, and her dedication; John Sterling; Maggie Richards; Elizabeth Shreve; Tracy Locke; and all of the Holt staff.

Special thanks to our mentor Dr. Irwin Goldstein, who not only supported and promoted us but also protected us from the wolves. He is both colleague and friend, a true inspiration and role model. He and the Urology staff at Boston University Medical Center were instrumental to our success. In alphabetical order, they include: Dr. Richard Babayan, Mary Chin, Karen Clements, Stan Ducharme, Karen Fink, Elizabeth Flaherty, Linda Frattura, Gina DiGravio and the rest of Boston Medical Center's corporate communications, Jean Kantey-Kiser, June Kevorkian, Dr. Robert Krane, Dr. Noel Kim, Linda King, Nancy Leahy, Laurie McCann, Scott Maitlin, Terry Payton, Dan Pollets, Dr. Abdul Traish, and Tiffany Werbin.

Also special thanks to the other teachers and mentors

who helped our lives and careers, particularly Dr. Cydelle Berlin, Dr. Natasha Kyprianou, Dr. Ron Moglia, Dr. Jacob Rajfer, Dr. Schlomo Raz, and Dr. Cheryl Springer.

Thank you, thank you to our family, not only our parents, but also our grandmothers, Jean Berman and Teal Friedman, our sons, Ethan and Max, and Jennifer's patient and supportive husband, Gregory Moore.

Thank you to our friends and colleagues, who lent us their moral and professional support: Dr. Helen Fisher, an inspiration and an advocate, as well as Kim Airs, Hope Ashby, Jeff Cottle, Carla Dionne, Stan Felder (along with the rest of the folks at Hisandherhealth.com, David Kitzmiller and Dr. Myron Murdock and team NEWSHE), Sandra Flowers, Jennifer Gilbert, Scott Goodwin, Dr. Susan Grant, Dr. Christine Hamori, Stephen Hulley, Dr. Gene Kelley, Dr. Roy J. Levin, Dr. Susan Love, Rachel Pauls, Lori Messenger, Dr. Cindy Meston, Dr. Abe Morgantaler, Nilou and Dr. Pedram Salmonpour, Dr. Marca Sipski, Susan Yarin, and Dr. Aline Zolbrod.

Last but not least, we'd like to thank our patients for sharing their stories for this book.

Index

Index

Frankel, Stephen, 194
Fred Hutchinson Cancer Research
    Center, 175
Freedman, Estelle B., 32
frequency of sex, 148–49
Freud and Freudian psychology, 27–28
future, the, 239–46

Galen, 22
Gay, Peter, 25
genitals, 41–42
    see also specific organs
Gerdes, Carolyn A., 83
Glaxo Wellcome, Inc., 124
goal-oriented approach to sex, 195–96,
    245
golden age and sexuality, 157–59, 169
Goldstein, Dr. Irwin, xi, 77, 80, 172,
    188
Goodwin, Dr. Scott, 75
Gorzalka, Dr. Boris B., 190
Greece, ancient, 21–22
group sex, 10
G-spot (Grafenberg spot), 48–49, 61,
    63–64, 152, 206, 212
    orgasm, *see* orgasm, G-spot
guanethidine, 89
Guttmacher Institute, Alan, 144
gynecological examination, *see* patient
    evaluation

Haldol, 90, 92
Hartley, Nina, 228
health:
    exercise and sexual, 185–92
    sex and overall, 192–94
heart, exercise's benefits for the, 189
heart attack, 94, 104, 159, 193
heart disease, 76–77, 107–8, 125, 159,
    175, 187
Heiman, Julia R., 204
helping yourself, suggestions for,
    195–219
hepatitis C, 34
high blood pressure, xiv, 77–78, 104,
    125, 175, 187
    medications for, 78, 89, 91
high-density lipoprotein (HDL), 78, 79,
    188
history of female sexuality, xiii, 21–36
HIV, 33–34, 137

homosexuality, 30, 134, 136–37
    lesbians, 137, 158, 181–82, 233
    sexual dysfunction affecting same sex
        couples, 181–82
hormonal problems, 80–85, 180
    see also specific hormones
Hormone of Desire, The (Rako), 113
hormone replacement therapy, 74, 81,
    100, 107–11, 157, 181
How Your Childhood Shapes Your Sexual Life
    (Zolbrod), 131
human papilloma virus (HPV), 34
Human Sexual Response (Masters and
    Johnson), 30–31
hymen, 46
hypertension, *see* high blood pressure
hypoactive sexual desire disorder, xii,
    13, 68, 69, 115
hypothalamus, 81, 135, 136
hysterectomy, xiv, xv, 73–75, 105,
    122
    problems after, 13–16, 242
    refining of surgery, 15–16
    total, 75
hysteria, 21–22, 24–25

impotence, *see* erectile dysfunction
incontinence, 88, 122, 156
Inderal, 89, 91
India, 33
infidelity, *see* extramarital sex
insurance, health, 219
Internet, sex on the, 242–43
interstitial cystitis, 87
*Intimate Matters: A History of Sexuality in
    America* (D'Emilio and Freedman),
    32
Isoptin, 89, 91

Japan, 33
Johnson, Virginia E., xv, 30–31, 54, 55,
    61, 63
Journal of the American Medical Association,
    xii

Kama Sutra, 23
Kaplan, Helen Singer, 55
Kaplowitz, Dr. Paul B., 135
Kegel, Arnold, 200
Kegel exercises, 64, 124, 152, 200–201,
    208

Index

Index

About the Authors

JENNIFER BERMAN, M.D., is one of the few female urologists in the country, with specialized training in female urology and female sexual dysfunction.

LAURA BERMAN, PH.D., has been working as a sex educator and therapist for more than a decade.

They appear regularly on *Good Morning America* and have appeared on *48 Hours*, *Larry King*, and *NBC Nightly News*. They have been featured in cover stories in *The New York Times Magazine* and *Newsweek*, as well as in *Redbook*, *Glamour*, *Cosmopolitan*, and *Harpers Bazaar*.

Formerly codirectors for the Women's Sexual Health Clinic at Boston University Medical Center, the Bermans are currently codirectors of the Network for Excellence in Women's Sexual Health (NEWSHE) and the Center for Pelvic Medicine at UCLA Department of Urology in Los Angeles.

ELISABETH BUMILLER is the author of *The Secrets of Mariko: A Year in the Life of a Japanese Woman and Her Family* and *May You Be the Mother of a Hundred Sons: A Journey among the Women of India*. She is currently City Hall Bureau Chief of *The New York Times*.